Alison Bowser is the ex-CEO of the Acne
Support Group and is currently working as an
independent healthcare consultant solely
responsible for organising a series of patient
rosacea education events around the UK. She
has recently qualified as a skin camouflage
practitioner and is a member of the British
Association of Skin Camouflage (BASC).

ACNE AND ROSACEA

THE COMPLETE GUIDE

ALISON BOWSER

Vermilion
LONDON

1 3 5 7 9 10 8 6 4 2

Published in 2010 by Vermilion, an imprint of Ebury Publishing

Ebury Publishing is a Random House Group company

The Random House Group Limited Reg. No. 954009

Addresses for companies within the Random House Group can be found at
www.rbooks.co.uk

A CIP catalogue record for this book is available from the British Library

The Random House Group Limited supports The Forest Stewardship
Council (FSC), the leading international forest certification organisation. All our
titles that are printed on Greenpeace-approved FSC-certified paper carry the FSC logo.
Our paper procurement policy can be found at www.rbooks.co.uk/environment

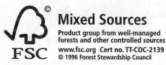

Mixed Sources

Product group from well-managed
forests and other controlled sources
www.fsc.org Cert no. TT-COC-2139
© 1996 Forest Stewardship Council

Designed and set by seagulls.net

Printed and bound in Great Britain by CPI Mackays, Chatham, ME5 8TD

ISBN 9780091929701

Copies are available at special rates for bulk orders.
Contact the sales development team on 020 7840 8487 for more information.

To buy books by your favourite authors and register for offers, visit www.rbooks.co.uk

The information in this book has been compiled by way of general guidance
in relation to the specific subjects addressed, but is not a substitute and not to be
relied on for medical, healthcare, pharmaceutical or other professional advice on specific
circumstances and in specific locations. Please consult your GP before changing, stopping or
starting any medical treatment. So far as the author is aware the information given is correct
and up to date as at June 2010. Practice, laws and regulations all change, and the reader
should obtain up-to-date professional advice on any such issues. The author and publishers
disclaim, as far as the law allows, any liability arising directly or indirectly from the use, or
misuse, of the information contained in this book.

The author and publisher gratefully acknowledge the permission granted to reproduce the
copyright material in this book. Every effort has been made to trace copyright holders and to
obtain their permission for the use of copyright material. The publisher apologises for any
errors or omissions in the above list and would be grateful if notified of any corrections that
should be incorporated in future reprints or editions of this book.

CONTENTS

FOREWORD

I first became interested in the area of psychodermatology when my cousin whom I was very close to developed the skin condition 'Vitiligo' as a teenager. I found it fascinating how profoundly a condition which was not believed to be painful or limiting in any way impacted upon her life, her decisions and even the way she saw herself. Like so many others who experience a skin disease, she began to be defined by it, to be stigmatised by it and to let it dictate her behaviour and even her quality of life. Over the years working in the area of psychodermatology, both as a clinician counselling patients and as a researcher writing books and publishing articles, I have seen this process enacted many times. Sadly the fact that the psycho-social effects often go unrecognized or are even minimized by some health practitioners means that, following a diagnosis, many people are left to fend for themselves when it comes to gaining practical information and support about their condition.

This is why I was delighted to provide the forward for Alison Bowser's book: *Acne and Rosacea: The Complete Guide*. This book provides not only insights and information for patients but it does so with a great attention to detail and a focus on the *experience* and development of the conditions over time.

The structure of the book and the reference to recent medical advances as well as the input from leading dermatology experts in the field makes it a useful resource, not only for the newly diagnosed patient but for anyone living with acne or rosacea at any stage of their illness. The book contains comprehensive information on treatments available for both dermatological conditions and answers many of the questions that patients often feel either too rushed or even too embarrassed to ask their doctors. It's important to note the fact that Alison Bowser herself lived with acne for many years as well as working for the Acne Support Group, and this is evident in the sensitivity and informative tone of the writing. The author succinctly, clearly and keeping medical jargon to a minimum presents recent research in the field and provides detailed insights on the process of living with acne and rosacea.

The holistic approach to describing and exploring both the physical and psycho-social implications of dermatological illness, which underpins this book, makes it valuable to both those living with acne and rosacea and their families, as well as health care professionals, including nurses and therapists working in dermatology settings. Alison Bowser has done a wonderful job in producing this book and I very much wish the work the success that it deserves.

Dr. Linda Papadopoulos
BA(Hons), MSc., PhD., CPsychol., CSci., AFBPsS

INTRODUCTION

Many people think of acne and rosacea as mild skin conditions, but anyone who has suffered from them knows the negative effects they can have on confidence and self-esteem. In most cases, acne and rosacea appear on the face – our mirror to the world – making it hard to hide away, unlike a patch of psoriasis on a knee or an itchy rash on the back. Cruel or even innocent stares can make someone with a skin condition on their face feel vulnerable and embarrassed. It's little surprise that having facial acne may cause someone to avoid eye contact and to send out the signal 'don't look at me'. These types of habit can become deeply embedded and affect confidence at the very time it may be most needed. Some have felt the best way of avoiding people looking at their face is to literally hide away from the world, locked behind doors that create a virtual prison.

Many people complain that they have never had their acne or rosacea explained. In addition, with all the mixed messages coming from skin-product marketers and 'beauticians' trying to sell you branded products, they don't know the best way to treat or care for their skin. They are often left bewildered and confused, feeling responsible for their skin's problems, which in turn leads to feelings of guilt.

I have written this guide to help anyone who has acne or rosacea, or knows or cares for someone with one of these skin conditions. It will take you, step-by-step, through a journey of discovery, helping you understand more about the causes and dispelling the myths. There will be tips on self-treating your condition, alternative treatments and everyday skincare. Specifically, I will help you overcome the negative emotions that these conditions can cause.

As a Chief Executive Officer of the world's only dedicated acne and rosacea charity, the Acne Support Group, I have helped over two million people with acne and rosacea deal with their condition. I also had over 12 years of life-affecting acne myself. My own acne started when I began high school and worsened year on year. By the time I left school I had already tried a wide range of antibiotics, creams, lotions and gels – and all seemed to have no effect. By this point I noticed it was spreading to my back and shoulders. I remember struggling to find corners within communal changing rooms in which to hide the horror of my ugly skin. I enjoyed swimming but this came to a gradual end as my confidence ebbed away. Each lesson required me to run from changing room to swimming pool in as few steps as possible. My acne became my main focus for nearly 12 years before I finally found the right treatment for me, but the decision to use it was not easily made. This treatment, called Roaccutane, is controversial and is discussed in depth later in this book.

My skin became so clear that, were it not for the scars left behind, I might have convinced myself I had imagined my years of acne. After turning this corner, I felt an immense sense of liberation and altruism – I wanted to shout from the rooftops that you didn't have to live with acne any more and help others overcome similar problems to mine.

Being involved with the Acne Support Group from its infancy meant I had a chance to shape its future. This gave me the opportunity to meet the country's top acne and rosacea experts in all areas of medicine, from dermatologists and doctors to nurses and pharmacists. I have campaigned for and against changes that would affect patients. There have been many successes and a fair share of failures, but all were worth fighting for, especially as both acne and rosacea have had a shockingly low priority for budgets, training and research. Working with a dedicated public relations consultant, Nula Bealby, meant we were finally able to put acne and rosacea into the public arena. The countless campaigns run through the Acne Support Group meant we could spread the word to an audience of millions. Being able to sit on the GMTV sofa and talk about the struggles of children with acne and the stigma of rosacea was among many of the fantastic achievements I would never have thought possible when I shied away from others because of my own embarrassing acne. It was liberating to discuss what had always been considered a taboo subject and to help people appreciate what can be done to turn their lives around, just as I had.

In writing this book, I hope to help even more people cope with their acne or rosacea. Containing some of the most comprehensive information available on acne treatments, it tackles controversial drugs head on to give in-depth advice that a doctor or nurse is unlikely to be able to provide in the normal time constraints of a consultation. I have drawn from my own experience and that of thousands of members of the Acne Support Group. There are contributions from some of the top skin experts in the UK, whose dedication and knowledge in the area of acne and rosacea treatments and research are considered to be among the best in the world.

Keeping medical jargon to a minimum and translating complex science into simple language, this guide is suitable for all ages, and for people with all types of acne and rosacea. It can also be used as a tool to help teachers, carers or healthcare professionals learn more about these skin conditions. No one needs to be kept in the dark about acne and rosacea any longer.

YOU ARE MORE LIKELY TO HAVE ACNE IF:

○ you usually have blackheads and/or whiteheads (small raised skin-coloured bumps)

○ you get spots on your face as well as your back, chest or shoulders

○ you are aged under 40

○ you have greasy skin

YOU ARE MORE LIKELY TO HAVE ROSACEA IF:

○ you have red patches restricted to your face

○ you experience blushing/flushing

○ you are over 40 (although it often affects younger people)

○ you get spots but not blackheads

You can read through this book or go straight to the chapters you feel are most relevant. If you have already started treating your acne, you are likely to have questions such as 'What is the best skincare for my skin type?' and 'Will changing my diet help?' Others may simply wish to understand if they are experiencing the first signs of rosacea and, if so, how to get the right treatments.

Quick Skin-type Quiz

If you are not sure which type of skin problem you have, the following easy-to-use self-assessment quiz will signpost you to the correct section of this book. This quiz does not replace a proper diagnosis from your own doctor.

You may already have a clear idea of your skin condition; perhaps you have received a diagnosis from your doctor or nurse. Many doctors agree that the signs of common acne are usually very difficult to confuse with other conditions. However, sometimes it is not so easy to be sure, especially if your skin has only just started to change. We also know that early rosacea can often be confused with common acne and may be treated as such by doctors. Treatments for acne may not always be suitable, with some of them being known to make rosacea worse, rather than better.

Start by circling each answer that applies most to you and add your scores up at the end. You may find your skin is better on some days than others, so choose the answers that apply to your skin on an *average* day.

1. How greasy is your skin?
A Dry/not very greasy
B Greasy
C Combination of both

2. Do you get flushing of the face?
A Yes
B No
C Sometimes

3. Do you get blackheads or whiteheads (see page 11)?
A No
B Yes
C Sometimes

4. Does your skin ever feel sensitive?
A Yes
B No
C Sometimes

5. Your age is

A Over 40

B Under 40

6. Do you have fair skin that burns easily in the sun?

A Yes

B No

Mostly As

You probably have rosacea. If you haven't already, visit your doctor for a diagnosis

See Part 2 of this book for all you need to learn about this condition.

Mostly Bs

You probably have acne (see Part 1 of this book for more information). Although it is not always necessary to check with a doctor, there are different types of acne, some of which may require prescription treatments from your doctor or a referral to a skin specialist (a dermatologist).

Mostly Cs

It's possible you may have both acne and rosacea, or a similar condition which requires a diagnosis from your doctor. Some of the conditions rosacea may be confused with are included in the section on rosacea. However, you may still find it helpful to read both parts of the book to learn more about general skincare tips and principles, and to discover how treatments commonly used for skin conditions can be used to maximum benefit.

PART ONE
ACNE

CHAPTER ONE
ACNE: WHAT IT IS AND WHO GETS IT

If you have acne you may feel reassured to know that you are not alone. This is one of the most common skin conditions in the world, with almost nine out of ten people worldwide[1] having it in a milder form.

You don't have to get lots of spots for it to be called acne – it's simply the name doctors give to many types of spots. Whether you prefer to call them spots, acne, breakouts, zits, pimples, blemishes or plukes is simply a matter of personal choice. This chapter will discuss all types of spots, from the mildest to the most severe, and the word 'acne' will be used to describe all of these.

What Causes Acne?

Acne is a common skin condition that starts with small blockages of oil in the hair follicle. There are four key components in the formation of acne:

○ Sensitivity to hormones
○ Sticky sebum

○ Abnormal cell growth
○ Bacteria

These four components usually work together to cause acne. However, not all four components may always be present, and they don't always occur in the same order.

Sensitivity to hormones

Acne can be caused by sensitivity to normal levels of male hormones in the body. We all have both male and female hormones, but it is testosterone (one of the male hormones) that increases the production of oil on our skin. The reason for this sensitivity is unclear, but it is likely to be connected to increases in hormone production triggered by puberty. As boys have greater quantities of male hormones, this would explain why boys can get more severe acne than girls. Hormone tests are rarely necessary for people with acne as the hormone changes that affect the grease glands are usually normal.

Sticky sebum

Sebum is another name for the oil or grease on our skin. Excess sebum is triggered by the hormone testosterone and will give the skin a shiny appearance. There may be a thin line between a 'healthy, shiny glow' and a greasy film. In people with acne, however, there is not only more sebum but it is also much thicker in consistency, which would be visible if you were to examine it under a microscope. This thickness makes it more 'gloopy' and viscous, a good sticky magnet for attracting anything around it.

People who have acne are more likely to have larger sebaceous (oil producing) glands than people who don't have acne, which could explain this problem of excess oil production.[2]

Abnormal cell growth

At the same time as this increase in grease production, the skin is also starting to slow down the rate at which it normally sheds dead skin cells. Although there is no good explanation for this, it is widely accepted that this is one of the factors in the causes of common acne.

All skin cells are produced at the bottom level of the skin called the dermis (the skin-making factory). These then grow and move up to make the epidermis, the upper level of skin. As they get closer to the top, these skin cells start to die. Eventually, the top layers – the visible skin we wash, scratch, put make-up on, stroke or pull – die and are shed with these everyday activities.

When there is abnormal cell production, not only are skin cells shed more slowly but there is a general increase in the amount of skin cells produced, compared with normal skin. You can imagine that this combination of increased skin cell production with the reduction in the rate that these skin cells shed is a recipe for a problem.

This abnormal cell growth causes a tiny blockage of the follicle. The follicle is the part of the skin that contains the hair. Attached to this follicle is the sac that produces oil, called the sebaceous gland. The oil produced in this gland escapes through the hair follicle and is released at the top. The blockage is described by doctors as a microcomedone, and is the starting point of acne. Now imagine that behind this blockage, grease is still being produced. As a 'plug' has now been formed by these dead skins cells, this oil has nowhere to escape; it can't just exit the follicle onto the skin as we might hope. This blockage may result in one of two things – either the oil behind the blockage becomes solid in texture (like solidified fat after a Sunday roast) and remains in the sebaceous gland doing little, or this grease starts to attract bacteria.

The first option, where the blockage remains solid, may appear on the skin in two ways. If the blockage of dead skin cells reaches the very top of the hair follicle and comes into contact with the air, it will turn dark brown/black. It used to be believed that this was because of contact with oxygen creating a chemical reaction, but more recently it has been found that the colour change is due to the skin cells that turn our skin dark (melanin). This is the classic blackhead most of us will be familiar with. However, if the blockage happens a bit further down within the follicle, just below the surface, it will push the skin up into a small bump. This is known as a whitehead. The whitehead often gets confused with inflammatory type acne (see page 12). It should really be called a 'skin-coloured head' but that doesn't have the same ring to it!

We have now identified what is known as non-inflammatory acne. This difference is helpful to know, as many treatments are aimed at one type of acne and not another. Most people will, however, have a combination of both types.

Bacteria

If the blackheads and whiteheads are non-inflammatory, what makes the spot inflamed? In an inflamed spot, the same process is going on within the skin – the tiny blockage, the excess grease described above. However, the difference is what happens to the oil when it is sitting in the follicle, trapped and with nowhere to go. Sometimes, this oil creates an ideal breeding ground for *Propionibacterium acnes* (known as *P. acnes* for short), the bacteria most commonly found in spots. These bacteria usually live on most people's skin doing no harm. That is, until they are given an ideal environment in which they can thrive and multiply, which is exactly what the blockage presents. There is no oxygen within this area, and this type of *P. acnes* bacteria particularly likes to grow without it. When these bacteria multiply, they will spread, causing damage around the follicle, rupturing it and attracting white blood cells whose primary job is to fight inflammation. To the human eye, this will now take on all the characteristics of the classic spot – yellow (which is how the white blood cells that fight infection appear) and red (which is caused by inflammation). The spot may be tiny or fairly large, and in some types of acne may be widespread and very deep. These are known as the inflammatory lesions of acne.

In reality, most people will have a mixture of both types of spot, but may be prone to getting one type more than the other. Some dermatologists believe that you must always use acne treatments that target the non-inflammatory type of blockages in order to stop the process which leads to the inflamed spots. More about the treatments later, but knowing which type of spots you have will be very helpful.

A study showed that 50 per cent of papules (red spots) arose from normal-looking skin (although a tiny invisible microcomedone may have been present); 25 per cent came from a whitehead (closed comedone) and the remaining 25 per cent came from a blackhead (an open comedone). This suggests that acne can be unpredictable.[3]

Life Cycle of a Spot

Even before a spot appears, things will be happening beneath the surface of the skin. For example, you may feel a slight tenderness, soreness or pain in the area just before the spot appears. However, it is fairly common for a spot to appear overnight. The type most likely to take time to appear will be the larger, red spots (papules/cysts); these may take a few days to enlarge and a few weeks to fade. Small pustules (yellow coloured) are the type most likely to appear quickly, sometimes within hours.

Understanding the different stages of a spot may help to reinforce the need to use anti-acne medications even when there are no visible spots. They work by attacking the causes of acne before they appear and are the best chance of keeping it under control.

Papule (red spot)

Stage 1

The very beginnings of a papule may occur up to three or four days before it is seen. The build-up of oil in the hair follicle will begin to mix with dead skin cells that make it sticky and viscous. This blockage leads to the beginning of an inflammatory response. At this stage, acne treatments would be able to fight inflammation and target the *P. acnes* bacteria, reducing the chances of it developing into stage 2.

Stage 2

The inflammation will now cause an area of redness and swelling, reaching the surface and becoming visible. This may occur two to five days from the first stage.

Stage 3

The papule enlarges as inflammatory responses increase its size and tenderness. After this, the spot will begin to die down and become a macule (a healing red spot). Stage 3 may last up to three weeks, although the average is seven days.

Stage 4

The skin is recovered. Some minor scarring may remain.

Comedone (blackhead, whitehead)

Stage 1

The build-up of dead skin cells in the hair follicle becomes trapped in the oil, as in a papule, but fails to attract the cells responsible for causing inflammation. This build-up may take several weeks.

Stage 2

If the blockage reaches the skin's surface it will turn black. Blackheads may last several weeks, months or even years if left untouched. The blockages that do not reach the surface and sit in the follicle (a closed comedone) may be very hard to notice with the naked eye; they are the type more likely to trigger an inflammatory response and turn into a papule. Research suggests that 25 per cent of closed comedones may resolve within three to four days, with 75 per cent developing into inflamed lesions.

Stage 3

If an open comedone is extracted, the pore may close over a period of a few days. However, some comedones may leave behind an enlarged pore due to being 'stretched' by the solid plug of the sebum.

THE ROLE OF GENES

Someone who had bad acne is more likely to have children who go on to develop acne, suggesting a strong genetic link. Research being undertaken at the UK's only dedicated skin institute, St John's, in London, is working at unravelling the mystery of why some people whose parents or other close relatives had acne go on to develop the condition. Studies carried out at the hospital have also looked at how twins go on to develop acne – in some cases, identical spots appear in the same place at the same time! The genetic link seems only a short time away from being proved.

Acne doesn't discriminate against age, nor does it target only some ethnic groups. Although it may be possible to identify those most likely to develop acne through their genes, we also know that anyone can get spots. Varying types of acne have different names to describe them, but all are part of the 'acne family'. The only people who may be less likely to develop acne are those living in remote tribes, possibly due to their 'undiluted' genes from lack of contact with the outside world.

Until the genetic key is discovered to unlock the secrets of acne, it is still important to treat acne at its earliest stages. This is especially important if the first signs of acne start very early into puberty (or just before), and if one or more of the parents had more than a mild acne problem when they were young. This could be an indicator of a more persistent type of acne that may need early intervention to avoid scarring.

Pustule (yellow spot)

Stage 1

Inflammatory responses in the hair follicle may be much faster than in a papule. It is difficult to estimate how long it may take the pustule to form, as this will depend on the size and depth of the inflammed area. If the inflammation is close to the surface of the skin, some pustules may appear within 10–12 hours.

Stage 2

If left untouched, pustules can heal into a macule within five days. Deeper pustules may last for up to two to six weeks before healing.

Different Types of Acne

Several different types, or variations, of acne exist; some are common while others are very rare. The acne most people have is also known as acne vulgaris (meaning common). Other types of acne are given different names to distinguish them from each other. The treatments vary according to the type of acne a person has (see pages 55–82). Types of acne can be divided into severity (how mild or severe they are) and different types. Some varieties of acne will have different degrees of severity, while others are only ever severe by nature.

Some doctors, when classifying acne, may wish to literally count spots in order to grade it. Doctors will usually divide acne into three different degrees – mild, moderate and severe – although there are also a few other common types. However, these descriptions are a helpful start to getting the acne correctly diagnosed and, most importantly, treated.

Mild acne

This describes skin that is beginning to show the typical first signs of acne: greasiness, open and closed blackheads and a few spots. Mild acne might be widespread or confined to one area. This type of acne is generally fairly easy to keep under control and will not be scarring. Although it is less noticeable than any other type, this does not mean that someone feels their acne is only a mild problem, nor that it shouldn't be distressing. The severity of acne does not always correlate with how it affects a person (see pages 241–2).

Moderate acne

As the description suggests, the acne will be more than mild. Again, it can be concentrated in one area or may be widespread. However, any spots may be larger, usually red and/or filled with pus with signs of open and closed comedones. Another factor that may distinguish this from mild acne would be spots showing various stages of the acne process, from newly formed spots, to healing spots and/or some scarring.

Severe acne

Truly severe acne is, luckily, quite rare. The usual signs of acne, such as red and yellow spots and comedones, will be present, but far more widespread and very angry looking. Someone with this type of acne will often have large cysts. A cyst is a pus-filled spot over 5 mm in diameter. It is usually very deep and may have a wide area of inflammation. This is the type of acne most likely to scar and needs to be treated with appropriate medication as soon as possible. Nodules are deep-seated, hard, lumpy spots. They may last for up to eight weeks. Some nodules may continue to return as it is difficult to remove all the contents. Squeezing nodules is never recommended as it is likely to cause scarring.

Severe acne can have quite a fast onset for some. To avoid permanent scarring, seek help immediately from a doctor if you have severe acne on any part of the body. Expect to return regularly (at least once a month) for close review. This condition will usually require a referral to a dermatologist (skin doctor).

Who Gets Acne?

The most common age to develop the first signs of acne – often greasy skin and blackheads – is early puberty. This is because the grease glands up to this stage are immature and too small to produce a lot of grease. Think about a child's smooth skin and how soft a baby's cheeks are – the last thing you would find with younger children is greasiness. So, for most, acne first appears around 11 years old or over. Girls are more likely to gets spots at a younger age because their puberty usually starts earlier than for boys. However, boys get more of the male hormones commonly responsible for increasing the grease output of the body, so they may be more likely to get worse acne than girls.

FAST FACTS
- 51 per cent of women aged 20–29 report still having acne.[4]
- Only 45 per cent of people with acne understand what causes it.[5]
- Fewer than a third of participants in a study with definite acne had sought help from a doctor.[6]

Acne can affect almost anyone, at any age. Luckily, for many teenagers the skin improves over time. Medical textbooks describe many varieties of acne, and some of these seem to affect certain age groups more than others.

Infantile acne

As the name suggests, this type of acne affects newborns and infants up to two. A newborn may have an acne eruption on the nose or cheeks. This is usually caused by a surge in maternal hormones that occurs as the baby is developing, and the outbreak typically clears in a matter of weeks, often without the need for any treatment. Many midwives or health visitors will describe these small spots as 'normal milk spots'. So, if these spots are fairly normal, when should a parent seek help?

If the spots have not cleared up on their own after four to six weeks then seek help from a doctor. There are a few treatments more commonly used on adult acne that can be recommended or prescribed and will often need to be used for a relatively short time. These will usually be products applied topically (on top of the skin). However, it is wise to start any such topical treatments by gradually introducing them to the tender skin of a baby. Using a damp cotton pad, apply the lotion or cream to the affected area, followed a few minutes later with a moisturiser such as baby lotion. This will help to reduce any dryness and keep the skin hydrated. If there is no improvement after a couple of months, then return to your doctor. Getting acne at this stage of life may require some further medical investigation if it doesn't clear after usual treatments. Similarly, if acne first appears at around three to six months without any previous signs, consult a doctor for further advice.

Childhood acne (ages two to six)

It is very rare for children of this age to develop acne, especially as the main cause of acne in newborns – the surge in maternal hormones passed on in the womb – will have disappeared. While the spots can be treated with usual acne treatments, the child will probably require a referral to a dermatologist if it fails to respond. Any possible underlying causes, such as problems with the endocrine (hormone producing) system or a tumour, could then be investigated. There are theories that getting acne at this age may be an indication of future acne that can be harder to treat and more severe in nature. Having the acne investigated and treated with stronger medicines at an earlier stage might help to avoid or reduce future problems.

Adolescent acne

This is by far the most common age to start developing acne. As it is so common, it should be considered more normal to have acne than not. As with acne at any age, if it appears to be getting worse or failing to respond to any self-medications, seek help from a doctor, nurse or pharmacist.

Adult acne

There is undoubtedly a group of people whose skin fails to improve following the more typical adolescent phase. Others may find their skin was relatively spot-free as a teenager, but becomes progressively worse in their 20s and 30s. For some, however, the first signs of acne do not appear until this age. This can often be more distressing than for those who have experienced ongoing teenage acne. Some people report how having acne for the first time in their late 20s was one of the hardest things they had to face, thinking they had somehow managed to escaped the scourge of most teenagers.

Up to 51 per cent of women have acne well into their 20s, but men are only just behind this figure. Some dermatologists estimate that 1 per cent of men and 5 per cent of women in their 40s are still affected by acne. The fact that there are more women than men in this age group may be a sign of an underlying condition known as polycystic ovary syndrome (PCOS). This is fairly common, occurring in up to 5 per cent of women.[7] Some doctors believe that any woman who presents with acne in their 30s should

WHERE ON THE BODY DOES ACNE APPEAR?

Acne occurs only where there are grease-producing glands (sebaceous glands). These are located on various parts of the body. The most commonly affected areas are:

- Face
- Neck
- Chest
- Back
- Shoulders

Some types of acne flare up on or around one area only, such as the scalp or buttocks. Other conditions linked to acne, but with different causes, can affect specific areas of the body where the skin folds, such as the groin, the armpits or under the breasts. Although it is possible to get spots in other areas of the body, spots do not occur on the soles of the feet or the palms as these areas have no sebaceous glands.

be considered for investigation into this condition. (For further information on PCOS, see Chapter 7.)

Senile acne

Although it may not be fair to consider anyone over 65 as 'senile', there is a type of acne that may appear in older people, taking the form of large blackheads. This will usually be painless and unlikely to cause any further problems, although doctors can treat these comedones with usual medication. This may also be a time when rosacea first appears, which may be confused with acne. Where it differs from senile acne is that it doesn't present with comedones. (Rosacea is covered in Part 2.)

> **TOP TIPS**
> ○ Only wash twice a day.
> ○ Use a soap-free cleanser.
> ○ A rough face cloth used twice a week can help remove excess dead skin cells.

Variations of Acne

Acne will usually have a fairly straightforward cause (see 'What Causes Acne', page 8). Some types, however, do not fit into the usual categories. Most of these are rare but include the following:

Acne conglobata

This type of acne usually affects more men than women and is most likely to occur between the ages of 18 and 30. It may occur on the site of an existing papule, pustule or comedone or on an area of skin previously affected by acne.

This rare and serious type of inflammatory acne requires aggressive treatment. Even with treatment, it may leave the skin scarred and permanently damaged. It is characterised by large cysts that are interconnected beneath the skin, forming 'tracts' or visible lumps that join one another. Even after clearing the pus-filled cysts and spots, it is possible that they will again become inflamed, resulting in the problem returning. This will usually occur in one concentrated area of the body, such as the buttocks. It is a painful and disfiguring condition, requiring immediate help from a dermatologist. Usually the strongest acne treatments will be given and, if necessary, a course of steroids will be prescribed.

Acne fulminans

This rare type of acne will be aggressive, painful and inflamed in a similar way to conglobata (see above). It can start very quickly and in some cases become severe in a matter of weeks. Where it differs is that it may present with painful joints and aches and pains similar to those experienced in arthritis. It can also be accompanied by a fever. This rare condition is documented in boys, rarely in females, and may be linked to the adrenal glands that release hormones. Its exact cause is not known. Acne fulminans can be treated with steroids, but will not usually respond to antibiotics as other types of acne will.

Hidradenitis suppurativa

This condition is linked to acne but affects only certain sweat-producing glands (apocrine glands). Unlike normal sweat glands which are triggered by overheating, the apocrine glands are triggered by stress, hormonal changes such as menstruation or sexual stimulation. It occurs in the armpits, nipples and the genitoanal region (the buttocks and genitals). Apocrine glands are stimulated by another hormone called adrenaline. This condition may be connected to acne because it is often found only in people who have had acne vulgaris.

The key signs of this condition are deep-seated nodules or lumps around the breasts, armpits or the genitoanal region. These may appear in isolation or in a group and the condition will continually relapse.

The lesions are made up of deep cysts and nodules with tract formation similar to conglobata (see above). Scarring is again common and secondary infection frequently occurs. This affects more women than men and is common in people who are overweight. If this type of acne fails to respond to aggressive treatments, it may be likely that the blockages will require surgery to help drain them. They will then be packed with sterile dressings and allowed to heal. This condition is very distressing and painful. Support is available from a dedicated support group (see pages 255–6).

Dissecting cellulitis of the scalp

This is similar to acne conglobata (see above) with the presence of nodules, cysts and interconnected tracks. However, when it is located on the scalp, it often leads to scarring; this in turn results in hair loss in those areas, and secondary infection may be common. This may respond quite well to steroid injections directly into the lesions, which can be painful and should be carried out by a specialist.

Acne mechanica

This might also be called 'friction acne' as it is often the result of anything that traps heat against the body for a prolonged period of time, or rubs or puts pressure on the skin. Any keen sportsman or woman who is also prone to acne may find that sports equipment pushed or held tightly next to sweaty skin, such as baseball caps, sweatbands and helmets, brings on a breakout in these areas.

Until quite recently, anyone with moderate to severe acne was disqualified from joining the armed forces. It was feared that tropical, humid weather conditions in war zones or practice areas might worsen existing acne on areas of the body where heavy armour or packs were worn in close contact with the skin. This ruling has changed, but anyone carrying heavy weights or equipment which is in prolonged contact with a sweating body should be aware that it can aggravate existing acne. In tropical areas, this can lead to potentially serious consequences such as the blood infection septicaemia, which can be life-threatening if not treated quickly.

It is not uncommon for acne to develop under tight bra straps, on the inner thighs or around areas of tight clothing that trap sweat. Even excessive phone use could, in theory, cause a similar problem. Maybe this condition could be called 'mobile phone acne'. This type of acne can be helped by reducing the pressure of tight clothing and carrying wet wipes to regularly remove excess sweat in the affected areas. Removing the sweat helps to reduce the problem.

Acne Majorca

This type of acne was first described in the 1970s when northern Europeans found that cheap holiday destinations such as Spain offered plenty of sun at affordable prices. Some people believe that sunlight can help their acne; indeed the UV light may well kill off the bacteria and sterilise existing acne. However, UV exposure also promotes a thickened, horny layer of skin. This layer can more easily obstruct the follicle of the sebaceous glands. The improvement in the skin is usually short term and lasts little longer than the tan itself. The result of obstructing the skin, however, is to make acne worse. In addition to this, oily suncreams and lotions can themselves cause an outbreak of acne. Always use acne-friendly brands that are oil-free.

Drug-induced acne

As the title suggests, some types of acne will flare up as a result of drugs taken either for other medical conditions or (illegally) for muscle-building effect. One mood stabiliser, lithium, will often trigger acne in patients. For those who need the benefits of a drug such as lithium, any resulting acne should be easy to control by taking anti-acne medication at the same time.

Steroids are used for hormone-related conditions but are also taken illegally by body builders who will commonly source them to help 'bulk up' their muscles quickly. They will often buy them from the internet or dealers. These might have the effect of building muscles quickly, but the side-effect of acne is common. Frighteningly, many will turn again to illegal sources to get powerful acne treatments that also have strong side-effects. People caught in this dangerous loop are risking their wellbeing for the sake of a sport.

Gram-negative folliculitis

This rare condition can easily be mistaken for acne vulgaris (common acne) because it occurs as the result of using long-term antibiotic medication to treat it. If people with acne experience a sudden flare-up after their skin has been clear for a while, and if they are taking a long-term course of antibiotics, gram-negative folliculitis should be investigated.

There are two types of gram-negative folliculitis. In 80 per cent of people, there will be superficial pustules without comedones that extend from the nose area to the chin and cheeks. In 20 per cent of cases, deep nodular and cystic spots will be seen (large, hard-feeling spots or softer red lumps, both of which are over 5 mm in diameter).

Treating this successfully can be very challenging, although some improvement is seen with isotretinoin (Roaccutane; see Chapter 3, pages 74–81). Clues as to whether you might have gram-negative folliculitis include:

○ You have used systemic antibiotics (antibiotics taken by mouth) for prolonged periods.
○ You have had a flare-up of pustular or cystic type spots and appear to be resistant to usual treatments.

Gram-negative organisms tend to be harboured in the nose, so testing for this condition will usually require a painless swab in the nostril. Sebum on the skin (the oiliness responsible for acne) provides an ideal moist environment for the bacteria to thrive.

Antibiotics often fail to solve the problem, possibly because they may kill the bacteria but have no effect on the sebum.

Acne in Pregnancy

Some women may experience a major flare-up of acne during pregnancy, regardless of whether they have had acne before or not. This is because the body releases a surge of hormones in early pregnancy, a mixture of both male and female hormones. Sensitivity to the male hormones (see pages 137–8) is responsible for breakouts, especially in the first trimester (three months). For the last two-thirds of pregnancy, the skin may improve and give the famous 'glow'.

The aim of caring for skin during pregnancy and breastfeeding is to maintain balance. However, regardless of whether the skin improves or gets worse, there are a few rules about how to treat the skin during this period:

○ If the skin is very greasy, wash with a soap-free cleanser as often as necessary.
○ It is safe to use a gentle exfoliator to unclog congested pores.
○ If your skin becomes dry, despite getting acne in some areas, continue to use skincare for combined skin types.
○ Use as much oil-free moisturiser as your skin needs.
○ Follow the skincare tips in Chapter 10.

Treating acne in pregnancy

Most of the advice in this section applies not only to pregnancy but also to breastfeeding.

If you are planning to become pregnant and are already using acne treatments, ensure you tell your doctor or nurse *before* pregnancy. If you discover you are pregnant after taking any medication to treat your acne, then make sure you tell your doctor, nurse or midwife as soon as possible. You will be advised on whether you need to stop medication or switch to a more suitable type for pregnancy. Some treatments are not recommended during this time, including certain prescription gels and creams. One of the few safe prescribed medications is erythromycin antibiotics, either in tablet form or used topically on the skin. Azelaic acid (prescription only), clindamycin and benzoyl peroxide are both considered safe to use during pregnancy. However, retinoid treatments, including gels and creams used on the skin, should be avoided until breastfeeding has stopped.

Choose any natural products with care and ensure they are not too oily. Although they may not be full of chemicals, they are not always advised during pregnancy. However, using aloe vera or the essential oils recommended later in this book, in particular tea tree and lavender, may be quite helpful (see page 97).

Just because you are pregnant, it does not mean you have to put up with acne. A good skincare regime and treatments recommended by your doctor should be able to keep outbreaks at bay.

CASE STUDY – SUE

When I first discovered I was pregnant, my joy quickly turned to despair as my skin literally started to erupt into the nastiest spots I have ever experienced. I guessed that it was because of my pregnancy, but it didn't stop me feeling very self conscious. It was bad enough for my doctor to mention it when I visited her early on in my pregnancy and she recommended a cream that I could use safely without harm to my baby. Although it wasn't brilliant, it did help and by the last three months of my pregnancy my skin was really getting a lot better – it seemed to change at the end into a very healthy glow. After my son was born I found my skin getting slightly worse again. I went back to using the creams, this time with an antibiotic treatment (I wasn't breastfeeding so I could use this safely) and my skin improved quickly. My advice to other women in my position is to ask for help from your doctor and don't worry – your skin will get better eventually.

A CHECKLIST WHEN VISITING THE DOCTOR OR NURSE

○ Remember to show all areas usually affected by acne, even if that means having to remove clothing. Make sure they take a look.

○ Tell them what your skin is like on a typical day, especially if your skin is looking quite good that day.

○ Ask about any medicine you are prescribed, especially if you have particular beliefs about certain types of medicine. There is no point being given a treatment if you know you are not going to take it.

Whatever the cause of your acne, there are still many treatment options available. The important thing is to understand why you are having problems and know how to treat the skin appropriately.

ACNE IN BLACK AND ASIAN SKIN TYPES

While we know that acne can affect anyone of any background or ethnicity, it is worth being aware of certain differences in skin colouring and what effect that can have on acne and, in particular, scarring.

Asian and black skin types are more prone to visible marks being left after a spot has gone. Although a healing spot is usually referred to as a macule, the dark pigmentation that remains is known as post-acne hyperpigmentation. As you might guess from the name, it is a deeper-coloured pigment, meaning the macule appears darker than the rest of the skin. This does not mean it will be permanent as many of these will heal well in time, but it can leave the skin tone looking uneven. This is different to pitted or raised scars because the hyperpigmentation is only a change of colour. When it is concealed (or skin camouflaged, see Chapter 11), it will not reflect the light at a different angle as pitted and raised scars do. There are a few steps to take to help if this affects you:

○ Use a camouflage concealer that matches your skin's natural colouring. This will help to blend in the colouring. This is suitable for men and women alike and results can be outstanding. (See Chapter 11 for more details.)

○ Azelaic acid can be a particularly helpful prescription treatment for darker skin types. This is because of the effect it has on the pigment.

○ If you use pomades or similar hair products, keep them away from the skin as they contain heavy oils and grease which are the enemy of acne. You can do this by using a towel or dry cloth to wipe the skin immediately after using the hair products.

CHAPTER TWO

GETTING YOUR FACTS STRAIGHT ON ACNE

Many explanations about the causes of acne are either untrue or based on old wives' tales. Some of these may have a minor element of truth but often get taken out of context or are blown out of proportion. Acne myths are often responsible for holding people back from seeking help, which might increase the chances of developing long-lasting or permanent scars, both physical and psychological. For example, a person might believe their breakout is due to their poor diet and feel too guilty to seek medical help. This chapter looks at the various questions people ask about acne, and examines the scientific evidence.

Is Acne Caused by Diet?

Many people have blamed acne directly on diet. The popular culprits are singled out as:

○ Chocolate
○ Sweets
○ Greasy or fried foods including chips and burgers
○ Snacks

O Cakes

O Milk

Given all the theories that link diet and acne, it is disappointing that there is little or no funding for robust scientific research to provide definite evidence, one way or another. However, recent research has revealed that two remote tribes, one in Paraguay and the other from Papua New Guinea, had almost no incidence of acne.[1] From examining their usual diet of fruit, fish, vegetables and nuts with little or no refined sugar or carbohydrates it seems plausible that their diet has influenced their skin. This may be easy to achieve in an environment where such food groups are relatively plentiful and make up part of society's everyday diet. However, it is worth remembering that other factors such as our genes may influence whether we develop acne; these tribes rarely move beyond their place of origin and therefore do not greatly mix their gene pools.

In a modern westernised diet where convenience foods are easily available, relatively affordable and give a quick energy hit, it takes a lot more discipline to stick to such a healthy diet. For this reason it could be useful to try a low-glycaemic index (GI) diet rich in any of the following food types:

O Wholegrain cereals

O Soya and linseed breads

O Most vegetables except parsnips

O Most fruits except dates and watermelon

O Whole-wheat pasta

O Brown rice

O Buckwheat

O Sweet potatoes

Theories about diet may also be connected to the changing relationship between parents and their adolescent children. At this time of life a parent may feel they are losing their influence on their child's diet, which may coincide with the first outbreaks of acne. It is easy to imagine a parent thinking, 'My child has their own pocket money, can buy sweets and chocolates, has become a faddy eater consuming vast quantities of carbohydrates – therefore their diet is to blame!' However, this may be seeking answers in the wrong place. If a child has no sweets or chocolates for a while does the acne improve? Given the evidence (or lack of it), we cannot answer this with 100 per cent certainty.

Perhaps the best advice when it comes to diet is to test the theories for yourself. To get a reliable answer, you have to be very strict and not cheat. Avoiding whole food groups, such as carbohydrates or dairy, may have other long-term or unwanted effects on your body, such as heart or immune system changes. The most sensible advice is to eat a healthy, balanced diet. However, it is unrealistic to expect diet to be a cure in itself, especially if the skin gets worse or develops signs of scarring.

Do Alcohol and Smoking Cause Acne?

Smoking and drinking alcohol are two vices commonly considered to be the culprits in acne. Evidence of a link to acne is scarce. However, it is worth considering that, as such habits generally affect our health, sleep quality and stress levels, they may have an impact on our immune system and ability to fight inflammation.

Research seems to offer conflicting results. One Italian survey studied women aged 25–50.[2] It concluded that 42 per cent of

IS ACNE CONTAGIOUS?

It is not possible to 'catch' acne or pass it on from skin-on-skin contact. Doctors have studied the effect of extracting the contents of a spot and injecting it directly into an unaffected area of the skin. This strange experiment concluded that it was not possible to spread spots.

Some people avoid kissing because they think they may get or pass on spots. This is rubbish – it's okay to kiss someone who has acne! It is also harmless to share towels or face cloths used for washing. Avoiding someone because of such fears only leads to increased feelings of embarrassment and awkwardness and is entirely unjustified.

women who smoked had acne compared with 10 per cent of non-smokers. They found that the smokers were more likely to have non-inflammatory type acne. However, sifting through several studies makes it impossible to draw any definite conclusions. A questionnaire sent to members of the Acne Support Group in 1997 found that 93 per cent were non-smokers. Theories about toxins in smoke causing blockages in the skin may sound credible but do not satisfactorily explain why, according to the Italian study, 58 per cent of people who smoke *don't* get acne.

Alcohol is reported to have an effect upon hormone levels; this may, in turn, have an impact on acne. Some studies have tried to prove a link between acne and excessive drinking but seem to give conflicting conclusions. Obviously, drinking in moderation should always be preferable to binge drinking, which is widely known to cause longer-term health and wellbeing issues.

Is Acne Caused by Dirt?

The myth that acne is caused by dirt is one of the more popular. This may be linked to the belief that the black of a blackhead is trapped dirt. We've already discussed how this colour is due to skin-colouring cells and nothing to do with being unclean (see page 11). In fact, some people who believe that dirt is a factor in their acne may be inclined to over-scrub the affected areas and risk making their acne appear worse. Some may feel so dirty they feel driven to use dangerous and inappropriate products to 'clean' their skin. Examples of these include neat household bleach, harsh scrubbing brushes or cleaning granules more commonly used to clean baths. Other measures include bathing or showering up to four times a day, using steam or near-boiling water directly on the skin or paying unaffordable amounts of money to have facials every week.

In a study that examined beliefs and perceptions about acne, 30 per cent of people believed their acne was related to poor skin hygiene.[3] This figure is worryingly high, especially considering there is no evidence to show this is true. Just because the skin has acne doesn't mean it should be treated harshly. Read the guide to washing in Chapter 10 for further advice.

CASE STUDY – SAM

I used to always go to the skin counter to try to find something, anything, that might work – whatever the cost. I would ask the beauty counter staff what would be best for my acne, which was pretty bad and very red. I always came away from the counter with a bag full of products and a crushed ego – the only way I can describe it was that I was made to feel as if I wasn't looking after my skin properly; I was doing something wrong. My skin was the cleanest you could imagine. I used to have two baths a day and literally scrub my skin raw because I felt so dirty. I would often hold back the tears as I left the beauty counter and stumble home praying that my new purchases would help me to feel clean for once. It never seemed to work. When a well-meaning beauty therapist suggested I needed to keep my skin clean it was the last straw and I lost my temper and shouted at her in frustration, 'I bet you my skin is cleaner than yours!' She looked startled. I realised then that I had to do something else to get rid of my acne. I visited my doctor who, luckily, seemed very clued up on the subject and reassured me that it was nothing to do with cleanliness. I still buy the beauty products, but I buy them for 'normal' skin types now and I make sure I don't ask for advice!

Is Acne Caused by too Many Hormones?

We have already covered the role hormones play in the formation of acne (see Chapter 1), but it is easy to misinterpret this as the body producing too many hormones. This belief leads many people to point the finger of blame solely at hormones. In reality, our skin has become sensitive to normal levels of hormones that circulate in the body. If it were a matter of hormones alone triggering acne, then because of significantly higher levels of androgens (male hormones) that men have compared with women, we would expect only men to get acne and not women. This, we know, is not the case. Some research has been carried out in this field and findings support the theory that there are no consistently higher levels of hormones in those with acne.

DOES MAKE-UP CAUSE ACNE?

Recent advances in cosmetics mean that fewer products contain harmful oils. Therefore, there is less chance of make-up having a direct link with acne. However, cheaper cosmetics may still have some oil content, which will usually be declared on product listings. Avoid oily products as much as possible and always remove make-up before going to bed. On its own, make-up is unlikely to cause major acne problems, and switching to oil-free brands will usually show immediate improvement.

Does Everyone Grow out of Acne?

Most people who get acne in adolescence find that it clears by the time they leave their teens.[4] However, it is not possible to predict who will or will not grow out of their acne. A minority may still have acne in their 20s, 30s or 40s, or even for most of their lifetime.

Of all the myths about acne, the belief that everyone grows out of acne can be the most unhelpful. If a person believes they may simply grow out of their spots they may not bother to seek treatment. Most adverts for spot creams and lotions are aimed at teenagers only but that doesn't mean it's a condition exclusive to them. If treatment is not sought or given long enough to work, it may lead to scarring. Scarring is the result of damage to the skin caused by a failure to treat acne. Don't let this myth put you off getting help or advising someone with acne to do so. Waiting to grow out of acne is pointless when there are so many effective treatments available.

ARE ACNE AND SPOTS DIFFERENT?

Acne and spots are the same. There is no medical distinction given by doctors between these words. However, some people mistakenly believe you need to have over a certain number of spots for it to be acne or that it has to be severe. Others seem to think that acne is only acne when you have been to see a dermatologist (a skin doctor). None of these are true. Acne, spots, whatever – it's all the same.

Does Stress Cause Acne?

There is some recent evidence that suggests stress alone may cause acne. This might be due to stress increasing the steroid hormone levels, which triggers acne. There is also plenty of evidence that acne can cause a range of emotions that include common signs of stress:

○ Anger
○ Changes in behaviour
○ Frequent crying
○ Difficulty in sleeping
○ Difficulty in concentrating
○ Anxiety

Particularly stressful times in a person's life, such as taking exams and getting married or divorced, can often make skin far worse. If you believe that stress makes your acne worse, seek suitable treatment right away. Take time to be aware of the stress triggers in your life and work out what you need to do to help you deal with that stress. One of the main effects of stress is the impact it has on sleep patterns. Many people who are stressed report feeling tired due to poor sleep. If you get stress-related acne, it is understandable to blame poor sleep and tiredness. Chapter 13 will help you to check if you might be suffering from depression triggered by stress or depression-related symptoms. If you feel worried, discuss these with your doctor. Luckily, for most people periods of stress will pass.

DOES TOO MUCH SEX GIVE YOU SPOTS?

While we know that acne most often first appears during puberty, there has never been any evidence to suggest that sexual activity (or thinking about it!) is responsible for acne breakouts. What we do know is that this time of life brings a change in body shape and sexual maturing, where one of the most common physical signs is the appearance of spots. This is a coincidence of nature, and nothing to do with sex.

Does Sunlight Improve Acne?

A suntan will often mask acne and work on the inflammatory factors in the skin to reduce the surface redness, making it look better. However, the quick fix that some people get from exposure to the sun hides a bigger problem; long-term exposure to ultraviolet light can prematurely age the skin and give a far higher chance of developing skin cancer in later life. Some people who believe that sunlight helps their acne risk their future health by using sun beds.

CASE STUDY – LOUISE

I used to start my holiday in the sun by burying my head in the sun bed and waiting until my back burnt. Then my skin would peel and after a few days it would look fantastic! Now I know so much about sun-damaged skin, I can't believe I did this. I make sure my husband keeps a careful check on my skin for any signs of moles. What was so ironic was that the acne on my back always came back worse after my tan had faded – so it was only a short-lived thing anyway, and I would end up more depressed than before my holiday! My advice? Don't bother with the sun – it's more dangerous than helpful.

See Chapter 12 for more information on sensible sun protection for acne skin types.

DOES PICKING ACNE CAUSE SCARS?

Most dermatologists strongly advise against squeezing spots. However, there are cases when, with only the gentlest of force and the cleanest of hands, it is perfectly acceptable to squeeze. The secret is knowing when not to. Chapter 5 explains more about the types of spots it is safe to touch and those to leave well alone. If you follow a sensible guide on how to do it, it is unlikely that you will scar. When a person forces, squeezes and pushes the skin (or even uses instruments such as pins, needles or tweezers) the risk of permanent scarring is most likely to occur.

Does Pregnancy Make Acne Worse?

Pregnancy doesn't necessarily make acne worse; in fact, some women find that their existing acne drastically improves. It is a matter of how the body responds to an increase in hormones that surge around the body to help the developing foetus. In the first trimester (three months), androgen levels are particularly high, which might be the reason some women experience a worsening of their acne; but as these levels equalise during the remainder of the pregnancy, the acne tends to do so too. The last few weeks often see skin give a positive 'glow'. However, if acne affects a woman at this time, it can still be treated. For information on treating acne during pregnancy, see pages 28–30.

Do Saunas and Steam Rooms Help Acne?

Both saunas and steam rooms make you sweat, which some people think will purge their skin. However, sweating actually traps in the dirt and can cause more harm than good; therefore, it is advisable that anyone prone to acne avoids both saunas and steam rooms.

CHAPTER THREE
ACNE TREATMENTS

When you consider how many myths there are about acne, it's not surprising so many people are unsure how to get the best from acne treatments. Much advice is given by well-meaning parents who may never have been given correct information themselves – and so the myths continue!

The good news about acne is that, for most people, it can be fairly straightforward to treat successfully. It can be very satisfying to see an improvement and to feel back in control of your skin. The goal of acne treatment is to stop new spots forming and to reduce any redness. Treatments are not, however, intended to reverse any existing scars or be a one-off wonder that needs to be used for only a few days. It takes persistence and determination to keep some acne under control.

FAST FACTS
- ○ The aim of treating acne is to stop new spots forming.
- ○ You need to give any treatment at least two months before judging it as 'good' or 'bad'.
- ○ Acne needs to be treated before scarring appears.

It's never too soon to start using treatments. Even a greasy complexion is a sign of acne and can soon cause problems if left untreated. Some people worry that products may end up doing more harm than good, but it is very rare that using spot products causes more problems than it solves. There is a combination of over 100 treatments that can be prescribed by a doctor, plus literally hundreds of over-the-counter products designed to help acne skin types, so there should be little excuse for acne to persist.

Getting the Most from Acne Treatments

For many people there may be some barriers in the way of finding success with treatments. The reasons for these failures may be put down to one or more of the following:

○ Lack of willpower or determination
○ Impatience
○ The effect of acne medication wears off
○ Using the wrong treatment for acne type

For a relatively small percentage of people, acne may last many years or even decades. If you just wait to 'grow out of it' or give up using treatments because you feel frustrated or disheartened, the only person that will suffer will be you. It's completely understandable to believe that giving up is easier than sticking to a medicine regime which requires patience and determination. However, having a strategy in place to counteract the above barriers might include:

○ Decide when you will use treatments to best fit in with your daily routine. You might connect taking or using your medication with other daily activities such as cleaning your teeth or putting in your contact lenses. If these are regular activities you can do without thinking about it, use this time to remind yourself to take or use your acne treatments.

○ If it helps, use a sticky note on your bathroom or bedroom mirror to remind you to use your medicine.

○ Use a diary to log when you can expect to give your skin a proper assessment, using the 'Two-Month Rule' (see pages 46–7). This will help ensure you are keeping your expectations realistic. Remember, the skin may go through many changes during the course of treatment, sometimes looking better, sometimes worse; but by two months any changes overall should be apparent. Be patient – no treatments work overnight, ever!

○ Take a minute to imagine how good it will feel to have clearer skin, and remind yourself of the benefits to you of taking or using your medication.

○ If you don't like tablets or using creams, don't get them! Tell your doctor or nurse which type of treatment you'd prefer before they prescribe you a treatment. If you walk away with a prescription for a cream that you know, deep down, you will not use then you will be wasting your time and money.

Over time, some people may find that the effects of their acne medication start to wear off, or that their results become erratic. It's worth being aware that skin will naturally have fluctuations when it may appear better some days and worse on others – just as we have good or bad hair days.

Sticking to a regime

This can be a challenge for people with acne problems, for all the reasons described above. It's natural to want creams or lotions to work instantly, and some spot cream manufacturers are keen to promote the idea of 'instant cures'. If only it were that simple! Treating a spot when it has appeared is already leaving it too late. Emergency or home-made remedies can leave the skin looking worse. If you can get to the earliest stages of acne, and help to stop the spot forming in the first place, then the skin will be more likely to show great improvement. So what can help you stick to a regime? The Two-Month Rule may help.

The Two-Month Rule

Despite some marketing campaigns, no treatments can work overnight or, worse still, instantly. While some treatments will soothe redness and help to make a spot look better, they will fail to get to the source of the problem. Helping to reduce the small blockages under the skin, which are usually the starting point of all acne, will help, but many 'quick cures' will not touch this aspect of acne. So how long is long enough? Use the 'Two-Month Rule':

Before two months
- ○ Try to estimate how many spots (on an average day) you have before starting treatment.
- ○ Whatever you use to help your acne – whether it is self-medication, prescribed acne treatment, home remedies or complementary therapies – try them as directed for a minimum of two months.

> ## WHEN **NOT** TO STICK TO THE TWO-MONTH RULE
> If your skin shows a sudden worsening in acne or if you develop an allergic reaction to what you are using (rather than a slight drying of the skin, which is common with acne creams and usually improves) then it is advisable to stop immediately. If the allergic reaction is severe, seek medical help straight away. If you have a mild reaction or a mild flare-up of acne, it may be worth persevering for a few more days to see if the skin settles; if it does, continue for the two-month period as suggested previously.

After two months
○ If you have more spots (on average) than you did before using the treatment you should change treatment.
○ If you have about the same amount of spots you should change treatment.
○ If you have less than half the average amount of spots then stick to the treatment and reassess in another two months.

This may not seem like a huge difference, but it is more realistic to expect a 50 per cent improvement than a 100 per cent clearance. When acne treatments are tested in trial conditions, improvement rates tend to be around the 50–75 per cent level. As yet, no known acne treatment has given a 100 per cent total clearance for 100 per cent of patients. The bottom line is, stick to treatments as directed and give them long enough to work.

CHOOSING THE RIGHT TREATMENT FOR YOU

There are two main categories of treatments:

○ Oral (tablets taken by mouth)
○ Topical (applied or used on the skin)

Some people may prefer one type over another. It's usually just a matter of preference. Some may prefer to take tablets every day because it cuts out having to rub on lotions, creams or gels. These types of topical product may burn, sting or tingle and even give off an unappealing smell. Others may choose to use these types, saying they prefer to keep medicine out of the body and use products directly on the areas affected. Often, however, the ideal treatment regime may be a combination of both types. If you have a strong opposition to using one particular type of medication, remember to tell your doctor or nurse before it is prescribed for you. If you are not sure what has been prescribed for you, then ask if it is to be used on the skin or taken by mouth. Many prescribers may not give the type of treatment a second thought until you ask. There are enough treatments to be able to give most patients a choice.

Beginning topical treatments

Anything applied topically to the skin has the potential to burn, sting, irritate, cause redness or peeling or produce an unwanted smell. While nobody would really rate these effects as desirable, they may often be a sign that the product is working. It is also fairly normal for new topical skin treatments to give a bit of a reaction. Give the skin a chance to grow used to products by trying the 'step-up' regime:

1. Start with using a small amount rather than 'slapping it on'.
2. If you are worried that your skin might react badly, then try testing in one small area only for a few days.
3. Apply to all areas usually affected, even when there are no spots to be seen.
4. Leave on the skin for up to 20 minutes.
5. After 20 minutes, remove gently with warm water on a cotton pad or with a gentle face wipe.
6. Apply oil-free moisturiser – as much as you feel your skin needs.
7. Start off applying at night only – this will allow any initial angry skin reaction to occur at night.

Gradually build up tolerance with this regime, increasing the amount of time the product is on the skin every week. This might be from 20 minutes to one hour, from one hour to overnight then from overnight to the full recommendations of the prescriber (this might be twice or three times a day).

Coming off treatments

When is the best time to stop using your acne medication? This will usually vary from person to person but a general rule would be to consider a gradual reduction in treatment to see if it makes any difference to the skin (unless directed otherwise by your doctor or nurse). You might, for example, have a prescribed gel or lotion that you use twice a day. When you feel you have reached a maximum level of benefit and your skin has fully improved, it might be wise to take a step-wise approach by reducing its use to

TIPS FOR USING TREATMENTS

Every product or treatment prescribed by your doctor should be used in the following way (with the exception of emergency spot treatments):

○ Apply creams or lotions to all areas usually affected by acne, not just the spots that you can see. Do this every time you apply creams or topical lotions directly onto the skin. Remember, the spots seen on the surface have probably taken a few days to form deeper beneath the surface of the skin.

○ Use treatments for a minimum of two months (see pages 46–7).

○ It may be helpful to use photos to decide if your skin is looking better, worse or no different. Take a picture before beginning treatment, making sure you can see the skin clearly enough. Take another photograph after two months. You are looking for a visible difference in the skin. Ignore spots that are healing or scarring. Bear in mind that skin may vary slightly each day, which may be influenced by factors such as the menstrual cycle, humid weather or lack of sleep.

once a day for two weeks. Then, if the skin is no worse after another two weeks, reduce it to once every other day for another two weeks. However, if the skin gets worse, then step back up again and maintain the dose that seems best for you. It will not be until you have stopped taking treatments that you will really know if they are helping any more or not. It is a matter of trial and error. This regime should be carried out under the agreement of the person who prescribed your treatment.

Stopping any treatments suddenly can result in the skin temporarily flaring up and seeming far worse. This is known as rebound acne and, as the name suggests, can make the acne return after a couple of days. Many doctors will not consider this possibility when they prescribe treatments, so ask about withdrawing in a step-wise fashion at the time of prescribing. If you are on more than one treatment for your acne, such as an antibiotic tablet and a cream, consider reducing the tablets first, in the way suggested above, before reducing the cream.

MYTHS ABOUT ACNE TREATMENTS

It's not just what gives you acne that is shrouded in myths. Treatments are just as likely to be a victim of well-meaning, but often futile, advice. By taking time to discover the truth about how acne treatments work, how to use them and how to manage any unwanted effects, it's likely that you will get better results. Let's consider the most common myths about treatments:

Myth: Slap on acne creams/lotions in double quantity on spots as they appear.
Fact: Applying more than is needed is likely to increase skin irritation and may over-dry the skin, which promotes more oil production and can make more spots.

Myth: If they don't work after three days don't bother; they must be rubbish.
Fact: Some spots may respond quickly to treatments, but as it takes several days for a spot to form this is not giving enough time to effectively work on the causes.

Myth: Any treatment that dries your skin out will make the problem worse.

Fact: Dryness is a cosmetic problem and can leave the skin feeling tight and uncomfortable. Some degree of drying will help remove the surface grease, which will reduce blockages in the skin and therefore be helpful. It's when the skin is over-dried that you will make it worse.

Myth: Antibiotics are bad for you because when you get ill in the future, they won't work.

Fact: There are many types of antibiotics and they work on a wide variety of bacteria throughout the body. By keeping antibiotics restricted to essential use only and by prescribing those that target the *P. acnes* most effectively, there is little chance of your needing those antibiotics to save your life in the future. The strongest antibiotics reserved for life-threatening conditions are not used for acne.

Myth: Some acne creams can cause skin cancer.

Fact: Creams are tested to decide if they might cause cancer in the future, and it is only if these studies show satisfactory results that a product can be licensed. Data from patients using creams are also used to decide if they are safe to continue to use; if they are not, they will be withdrawn from the market based on evidence of harm.

Myth: Treatments that doctors give will cause you more harm than good.

Fact: Some people hold certain beliefs about medicines causing harm to the body. Everyone is entitled to their own beliefs and may wish to avoid medicines for this reason. However, careful steps are taken to ensure that all medicines prescribed are as safe as possible.

Myth: You have to treat from the inside first.
Fact: Acne can be just as effectively treated from the outside (using creams) as it can from the inside (taking tablets). There is no particular evidence to suggest one is better than another.

There are probably many more myths, but these give you an idea of the common concerns that might hold a person back from really giving their treatments a chance to work.

Golden rules of treating acne

When it comes to treating acne, there are a few golden rules that will help ensure you get the maximum benefit. These are so simple that if everyone followed them, most people with acne would find their skin improved. When acne starts to clear up, not only does it improve confidence, but it also reduces the chances of developing scars that may last a lifetime.

1. Always use treatments as prescribed or directed. Take time to read the leaflet that comes in the medicine packet. If you need any further help ask your doctor or pharmacist.
2. Apply topical treatments on *all* areas usually affected, even when you can't see any spots or blackheads.
3. Use the 20-minute wash-off rule (see page 49).

4. Use treatments for at least two months before you start to judge how well they are working (see pages 46–7).
5. Some treatments will need to be used for a period of many months or as long as your skin is in a state of acne.
6. Avoid suddenly stopping acne treatment as this may cause 'rebound' acne (when acne gets worse, see page 51).

TOP QUESTIONS TO ASK ABOUT YOUR TREATMENTS

○ How do I use this medication?
○ What side-effects might I expect?
○ What sort of improvement can I expect?
○ What else can I use if this doesn't' work?

By sticking at acne treatments for long enough and using the right amount of treatment exactly as prescribed, you will greatly improve your chances of keeping in control of your skin. However, if your skin becomes progressively worse over a period of a few weeks, or if you experience any unwanted side-effects, then you may need to consider changing treatment.

FAST FACTS

Side-effects of medication can be very common and will usually reduce over time as the skin becomes used to it. If, however, you notice any extreme or unexpected effects, contact your doctor or pharmacist immediately. You can report a side-effect of your medicine at www.mhra.gsi

First-line Treatments

These are treatments you can buy without a prescription.

Self-medication

You, as the consumer, can choose what you wish to purchase and can do so without any restrictions. These will usually be first-line treatments that can be used as soon as the skin starts to show signs of acne. They can be purchased from various suppliers, including herbal or homeopathic practitioners, the internet, beauty salons, supermarkets and pharmacies. However, do ensure that any treatments you buy online are from reputable websites.

What you seek in a treatment should depend upon how bad (severe) the acne usually is. The odd spot on an otherwise acne-free skin type could be treated with emergency spot remedies that can be dabbed on. These will reduce surface redness and calm the spot, helping to speed up healing. However, be aware that such products should not be used on broken skin, or for ongoing anti-acne use in the place of other treatments designed to be used on a long-term basis.

Milder acne problems can be helped with a selection of products that come in a variety of formulations such as wipes, masks, cleansers, pads and strips. Often deciding which to use is merely a matter of preference and budget. Try to avoid using too many at once as using more does not mean skin clears faster.

Usually the first place to go for self-help treatments would be the pharmacist or supermarket. For mild acne start with a wash designed for acne skin types. For blackheads and blocked skin, try products that have an exfoliating action on the skin. Exfoliating is when the top (dead skin cell) layers are removed either by the action of a rough cloth or by products containing something that will have the same abrasive action. More advice on skincare can be found in Chapter 10.

A SIMPLE GUIDE TO SELF-HELP TREATMENTS

○ Emergency spot treatments will target redness and inflammation and may soothe the skin.

○ Anti-spot products need to work on at least one of the four main causes of acne (see Chapter 1). They might affect abnormal cell growth, for example, or target the bacteria.

○ There is an extensive range of washes, exfoliators and skincare products that can be used at the first signs of acne and will be suitable for most skin types (sensitive, greasy and so on). These are usually an excellent starting point.

Key acne-fighting ingredients

Look for products aimed at greasy, acne-type or spot-prone skin. These ranges will usually include ingredients that help reduce redness and remove surface skin cells in an exfoliating action.

Benzoyl peroxide (BP): One of the oldest and still most effective ingredients, this chemical attacks the bacteria that cause spots. In order to thrive, bacteria require an oxygen-free environment, which is why the blocked pore is such an ideal breeding ground for acne. However, where BP steps in is by introducing oxygen into the follicle. This oxygen helps to kill the bacteria and reduces redness. Many prescription acne treatments still contain this useful ingredient, and many dermatologists firmly believe in its benefits in helping mild to moderate acne. The other main advantage of BP is that it prevents the development of antibiotic resistance.

Despite its usefulness in treating acne, be aware of two key problems with BP:

○ It is likely to cause excessive drying and/or redness of the skin.
○ It won't bleach your skin but it will bleach anything else it comes into contact with. That includes hair, eyebrows, towels and bedding. Use old towels or bed sheets to avoid mishaps.

BP is available in different strengths between 2 and 10 per cent. Some studies have compared these different strengths. The results suggest that using the lowest percentages (2, 4.5 or 5) gives the same results as the higher (10). The advantage of sticking with the lower strengths is there will be less chance of experiencing unwanted effects such as tingling, redness, dryness or irritation.

A wide range of acne creams/lotions and washes contains BP. Take a careful look at the ingredient list and note the percentage. If there is a choice of percentages, try the lowest first. You can always move up in strength if you feel you need to later.

Salicylic acid: This common ingredient can also be found in aspirin and wart treatments. It works very well as a natural exfoliator. By removing dead skin cells it reduces blockages within the skin that cause blackheads to form.

Don't be put off by the word 'acid' as this doesn't mean it will melt the skin away. This type of product is commonly found in a wide range of skincare products especially formulated for greasy, spot-prone skins, and may come in different strengths. You can find it in washes, cleansers, pads and lotions. It is even added to make-up and coversticks.

Used on its own it is unlikely to solve anything more than a mild acne problem, but it can be useful as part of a skincare regime at the same time as treating your skin with prescription products. Like benzoyl peroxide it can be drying, but applying an oil-free moisturiser afterwards will help. Some skincare products contain only the lowest amount of salicylic acid, so try to find those with a higher percentage (5 per cent or more).

Be aware that it should not be used by pregnant or breast-feeding women. This also applies to women who are likely to become pregnant. If you are allergic to aspirin, then you should not use salicylic-containing products.

Other self-medications

As long as you stick to the 'Two-Month rule' (see pages 46–7), you can try a range of self-medications from the pharmacist or supermarket. Many of these will be marketed at teenagers but are not exclusively for teenage skin. Brand names aside, many of the ranges available off the shelf will contain the same basic range of ingredients, which may or may not include benzoyl peroxide or salicylic acid. There are other ingredients that may help reduce bacteria or blocked pores or both. The current list is extensive and the choice is down to individual preference and budget. However, bear in mind three things:

○ Evidence they work may be minimal – few or no studies may have been done to compare them against other proven treatments.
○ Often the same key acne-fighting ingredients are available in the same brand range but in different strengths. If in doubt, start with the mildest first and work up.

○ Do not wait for these types of treatment to work if your skin seems to be getting progressively worse or scarring (remember the Two-Month rule).

When Should You Visit a Doctor or Nurse?

Usually it would be advisable to consult your doctor when:
○ You have already tried at least two different types of self-medication.
○ Your skin is getting worse or failing to improve.
○ Your skin is starting to scar.
○ You feel very distressed about your skin and unable to carry on with normal daily activity because of how you feel.

It is perfectly acceptable to treat your acne using self-medications (see above). However, if your skin is not improving after using treatments for at least two months, then speak to your doctor or nurse who will be able to prescribe from a wide variety of acne medications. Deciding which type is most suitable for you will depend upon the type of acne you have (mainly inflammatory or non-inflammatory, see pages 11–12).

Many doctors and nurses see patients with acne regularly and are confident and up-to-date with the latest advances in acne treatments. Others, however, may appear less interested or have less experience. If you belong to a group practice where more than one doctor is available, ask the receptionist if any of the doctors or nurses have a special interest in dermatology. This might help to identify those most able to assist before you realise your own GP doesn't really know as much as their colleagues.

Once you have identified your preferred doctor or nurse, bear in mind that acne is a visual condition. Therefore being able to see the skin well, under a good light, is usually necessary. While a doctor will probably think nothing of asking you to sit under a glaring light without make-up (or camouflage if you are a man), it is understandable to feel self-conscious. Some tips to make your visit to the doctor easier include:

○ Request the first appointment of the day to allow you to slip in and away before the waiting room becomes too full. Alternatively, the last appointment available might mean there are fewer people around.

○ If you wear make-up or camouflage, bring your remover with you and be prepared to take it off in front of the doctor if necessary. Bring extra make-up to reapply if you need to before you leave the surgery.

○ If your skin is prone to having 'good' and 'bad' days, you can usually guarantee it will be fairly good on the day you visit your doctor. To ensure they understand what your skin looks like on a *typical* day, take some photographic evidence. With mobile phones and digital cameras, you'll never need to print them off. Again, remove any make-up before snapping your picture.

These strategies will show your doctor or nurse how seriously you take your acne, and in turn, how seriously you expect them to take it. Remember to tell them what medications you have already tried or currently use, including any self-medication.

Your doctor should take your acne seriously. It is usual for them to assess your skin, make a note of any treatments you have already used and then suggest a treatment based on these factors.

Just because your acne is not life-threatening doesn't mean it should be ignored or trivialised. If you feel you are not being taken seriously, consider if you have been clear in telling your doctor:

1. **How your skin makes you feel**. You may not be a person who likes to share their feelings with a stranger, but even telling them how acne affects your life or daily activities such as socialising, going to school or work will let them understand its impact. This may make a difference to the type of treatment they recommend.
2. **If anyone else in your family has had acne**. If a close relative has had a problem with acne, then it may be that you are going to have a more persistent problem than some (see page 15). Acne that seems to be hereditary may end up being harder to treat, slightly more aggressive and likely to lead to scarring, especially if it started at a particularly young age.
3. **What else you have used**. This is important to share, especially if you have tried products containing benzoyl peroxide.

CASE STUDY – RUBY

I found it really difficult to talk to my doctor about my skin. By the time my appointment came through my skin would usually be looking a lot better, which was really annoying because I had the feeling the doctor thought I was making it up! When I went last time, I wanted her to take me seriously so I showed her the pictures of my skin I had taken on my mobile phone the previous week when it was really bad. I also booked the last appointment and took my make-up remover with me to show her my skin. It was quite funny really because the doctor told me that she

CLASSIFICATIONS OF UK MEDICINES

In the UK, the Medicines and Healthcare Products Regulatory Agency (MHRA) is responsible for licensing and classifying all medicinal products including, more recently, herbal remedies. Some treatments might be considered to have more risks than others, or contain ingredients that require a suitably qualified doctor, nurse or pharmacist to make a decision based on your individual health and health history before they can be prescribed.

Next to each type of treatment listed below is a code: GSL, P, POM or HOM. These abbreviations represent:

General Sale List (GSL): These drugs can be sold with reasonable safety without the supervision of a pharmacist, for example in a supermarket. However, they can only be sold from lockable premises and in the original manufacturer's packs.

Pharmacy (P): Pharmacy medicines do not require a prescription. They may be sold or supplied only in a registered pharmacy by or under the supervision of a pharmacist.

Prescription Only Medicine (POM): These medicines may be sold or supplied only from a registered pharmacy and in accordance with a prescription issued by an appropriate practitioner (a doctor, dentist, nurse independent prescriber, pharmacist independent prescriber or supplementary prescriber).

Hospital Only Medicine (HOM): These can be prescribed only by or under the supervision of a hospital doctor.

thought my skin looked much worse with my make-up off yet my foundation on it looked really natural. She complimented me on disguising my skin problem so well and asked me where I had got my foundation from! Once she could see it close-up, and especially after she looked at my photos, she agreed that what she had been prescribing wasn't strong enough for me. She changed my treatment and six weeks later my skin is already looking 100 per cent better. Fingers crossed it will stay that way. I still wear my foundation but I know that underneath it my skin is already so much better than it was.

Second-line Treatments

Second-line treatments are those that are usually prescribed by a doctor or nurse after trying self-selected treatments from a pharmacy or supermarket. They will usually contain ingredients licensed to be prescribed only by a health professional.

Nicotinamide (P or GSL)
This is part of the vitamin B group (B3) and has an anti-inflammatory effect on the skin. It can either be prescribed or purchased from a pharmacist. Some patients report that it is very well tolerated on the skin. This is marketed as Freederm®.

Topical retinolds (POM)
The chemical name is tretinoin or isotretinoin; both are similar and based on vitamin A. However, vitamin A creams alone will not achieve the same results as they would need to be used in very high doses, and vitamin A is difficult to keep stable without it 'going off' quickly.

This type of treatment has an effect on the development of skin cells and is therefore used in conditions where the hair canal in the skin is blocked or plugged. Its major effect is on the non-inflammatory lesions of acne (blackheads and whiteheads). With regular use it causes softening and expulsion of the blackheads and helps to prevent them reforming.

As retinoid creams and gels can also cause sensitivity to sunlight, always apply a sunscreen if using them on the skin during the day. If you have been advised to apply it once a day, try using it at night to reduce the exposure to UV daylight.

Adapalene (POM)

This topical gel is not exactly a retinoid but is chemically similar. It can be very helpful on both inflamed and non-inflamed acne. Some patients report that it causes less irritation than some other prescribed topical creams.

Topical antibiotics (POM)

The most commonly used topical agents include the antibiotics tetracycline, erythromycin or clindamycin. These are usually present in an alcoholic solution. They are sometimes mixed in a more soothing lotion or gel format. If you know you would prefer a gel to a lotion, tell your doctor or nurse before they give you your prescription.

They work by reducing the level of bacteria in the skin, while also reducing inflammation commonly present around the spots themselves. They are particularly useful in mild to moderate acne. The antibiotic should be applied twice a day (or as otherwise directed) to all affected areas. Topical antibiotics when used alone have little direct effect on the non-inflamed type of spots (blackheads and whiteheads) so if you have the non-inflammatory type of acne as well, ask your doctor or nurse to prescribe something else in addition to help the blocked pores.

In general, antibiotics are very well tolerated by the skin and have few side-effects. Scientific research has proven that applying antibiotics to the skin can be as helpful as taking them by mouth.

UNDERSTANDING MORE ABOUT ACNE MEDICATIONS

This is a combination of over 100 treatments currently available on prescription from your doctor. Some of these will be branded products, meaning they will be given a brand name by the manufacturer and marketed under this brand name. An example of this is the drug known as Duac®. This is the name given to the brand, but the generic name is benzoyl peroxide 5% and clindamycin 1%. As brand names change from time to time, this book will focus on the generic name of the drug. The generic name will always be included in the medicines information leaflet, also known as the patient information leaflet, that comes with your medicine. This includes those medicines you may have purchased from a supermarket or pharmacy. Many people don't bother to read this information, but it is worth taking a few minutes to read through the leaflet to help you understand:

○ the possible side-effects you might experience
○ what the medicine has been prescribed/licensed for
○ how the medicine might interact with other medicines or supplements you might be taking
○ how to take the treatment to get the maximum benefit from it

It is common for doctors to mix treatments to give the maximum benefit from a variety of key ingredients. This combination may be a mixture of antibiotic tablets with a cream to use on the skin at the same time.

Combined topical antibiotics (POM)

To boost the benefits of antibiotics, some companies have developed acne treatments that combine them with other anti-acne ingredients. These are clinically proven to be better than single active ingredients alone. The added ingredients are one of the following:

○ Benzoyl peroxide (BP)
○ Zinc
○ Tretinoin
○ Adapalene

Azelaic acid (POM)

This comes in a cream formula. While it was prescribed quite commonly in the past, it is not very popular as an acne treatment now, and tends to be used in those who have not responded to other treatments. Azelaic acid works well both as an antibacterial treatment and to help reduce the build-up of dead skin cells. It is not an antibiotic so it doesn't have the problem of patients becoming resistant to it. As it also targets melanin in the skin, it can be very useful in those who develop post-acne pigmentation (darkened patches of skin colouring). Darker skin types are most likely to develop this type of pigmentation problem, so it is worth asking to try this treatment if you fit into that category.

Zinc sulphate (GSL)

Zinc sulphate capsules at a dose of 220 mg three times a day is a rather old-fashioned treatment for acne but can be quite helpful. The zinc may be used in combination with antibiotics (see above) to improve the effect. It has been shown to promote healing of wounds, such as leg ulcers, but the exact method by which it works in acne is unknown.

Zinc may cause stomach upsets and possibly nausea or diarrhoea. New effervescent preparations seem to help reduce these symptoms. Zinc is also the ingredient in one of the topical antibiotic preparations, with studies suggesting it gives a boost to the antibiotic, helping to reduce resistance[1]. An explanation for this seems hard to find as the way that zinc works in the skin is still not fully understood.

Antibiotic Tablets

Some doctors or nurses prefer to prescribe tablets for treating acne. Likewise, some people prefer to take medication by mouth. More recent prescribing guidelines support the use of both topical and oral treatments together. There are many types of antibiotics that are particularly useful for treating acne. As a general rule, these should be given for a period of time, usually no less than six months.

The most common types of antibiotics used are: tetracyclines (of which minocycline is one), erythromycin, minocycline and trimethoprim. These fight the bacteria present in inflamed acne and also reduce redness and swelling. They will not, however, help with the non-inflamed type of acne and should therefore be taken at the same time as using topical gels, creams or lotions more suitable for this type of acne. Antibiotic tablets don't help blackheads or whiteheads.

Taking antibiotics correctly

Taking some types of antibiotics properly may require swallowing them on an empty stomach. To ensure the maximum benefit, tetracycline or oxytetracycline should be taken one hour before food and two hours after last eating. Tetracyclines may also be affected by milk, including milk in foods or drinks such as tea or coffee. If you have erratic eating habits, ask the doctor or nurse to ensure that the antibiotic they prescribe isn't affected by food or drink.

Some antibiotics may reduce the effectiveness of the contraceptive pill for a few weeks when you first start the course. If you are currently taking the pill you should discuss this with your doctor if there is a possibility of your becoming pregnant. It is not unusual to experience some degree of stomach upset when taking antibiotics, especially with erythromycin. If they affect you in this way, then talk to your doctor, especially if you are taking other medications such as the pill.

Tetracycline

The usual recommended dosage of oxytretracycline is 1 gram a day. This will usually mean you will need to take up to four tablets in one day. Sometimes it will be given in two 500 mg doses, but as the antibiotics do not last long in the system, you may need to space the time out evenly between taking them. If minocycline is being used the normal dose is 50–100 mg a day, and doxycycline, which also falls into this category, is taken at 100 mg a day. Another type of tetracycline is called lymecycline (Tetralysal®), which is prescribed at a dose of 408 mg once daily. It is claimed this antibiotic is better absorbed by the body and is not affected by consuming milk or milk products.

There are reports of increasing resistance to the *P. acnes* so it is better to use most antibiotics in this group in conjunction with other anti-acne products that don't contain antibiotics.

Erythromycin and clindamycin (macrolides)

Erythromycin is often prescribed for inflammatory acne. It is considered to be safe to use in pregnancy and during breast feeding and is therefore used in preference to the tetracyclines by some doctors for women of childbearing age, or even during pregnancy and breastfeeding.

Like oxytetracycline, erythromycin should be started at 1 gram a day – two daily doses of 500 mg.

Clindamycin is an antibiotic which is not commonly used to treat acne, but may still be helpful. In low doses, the chances of developing side-effects are reduced. However, if you experience diarrhoea, then you should consult your doctor urgently because it can cause colitis (inflammation of the gut).

Trimethoprim

Trimethoprim can also be used to help acne and is usually prescribed at doses of 400–600 mg a day, taken in divided doses. It is very effective in acne and used by many dermatologists, but it is not technically licensed for treatment. Some people feel sick when they take this medicine and may develop unwanted side effects such as a rash. If this happens to you, consult your doctor immediately.

Antibiotic resistance

For the last few decades, antibiotics have remained the most commonly prescribed agent for treating acne. Many millions of prescriptions for oral antibiotics are dispensed a year.

Various studies are showing how increasing numbers of patients are becoming resistant to antibiotics. One study reported in the *British Journal of Dermatology* suggested that up to 51 per cent of 4,724 patients had shown resistance. With the increasing rate of antibiotic resistance, this figure is likely to grow even higher. Many researchers and scientists who study microbiology report their fears over the widespread use of antibiotics. They are urging doctors and nurses to rethink current acne treatment policy of using antibiotics so readily.

Other studies seem to show a similar pattern of resistance that is growing steadily as more antibiotics are prescribed. This resistance applies to either tablets or creams/lotions and gels applied to the skin. Anyone taking any type of long-term antibiotics (four weeks plus) will have an increased risk of developing a resistance to them. Resistance can happen in a number of ways and to some antibiotics more readily than to others. One of the types most likely to result in resistance is erythromycin, followed by tetracyclines.

If your bacteria have become resistant to certain types of antibiotics, your acne may get worse. A way you might notice this is if you notice that taking your antibiotics no longer seems to help your skin, or alternatively if they fail to work at all, despite taking them correctly and giving them long enough to work. If this is the case, make a note of the name of the antibiotic and tell your doctor or nurse so they can record that you are no longer responding to it. Be aware that doctors don't always routinely make a note of this, so prompting them to do so might help you next time you need an antibiotic.

It is possible to spread the resistant bacteria to other people through everyday close contact. This might be in hugs or cuddling when there is skin contact. Microbiologists have noted that this contact can result in the other person also becoming resistant to the same antibiotic. This can be seen more in siblings and could explain why a certain antibiotic fails to work, despite the patient taking it as prescribed and never having taken it before.

Further studies on bacteria have resulted in some simple guidelines to how this resistance can be reduced. Following the 'golden rules' below will help.

GOLDEN RULES OF TAKING ANTIBIOTICS

○ Always complete the course. By failing to finish a course, or by simply taking a tablet on a 'when I remember to' basis, it is possible to increase the chance of the *P. acnes* becoming resistant, as well as not giving them enough chance to work.

○ Use benzoyl peroxide (BP) as a 'wash-out' at least once a week (see self-medication section, pages 56–7).[2] In laboratory tests, the BP works by eliminating the resistance, making some experts recommend that every person taking antibiotics for their acne should also use BP at least once a week.

○ Never share your antibiotics with anyone else as it may cause unwanted side-effects.

○ Doxycycline is the antibiotic most likely to make the skin very sensitive to sunlight (phototoxic). Use a good, oil-free sunscreen if using this, even in cloudy weather.

○ Tetracycline antibiotics are not suitable for children under 13 or pregnant women as they can cause staining of the teeth and bone development problems.

Contraceptive Pills

In women who require contraception, the combined contraceptive pill can be used without problems for those who have acne in the majority of cases and it can significantly improve acne. However, the mini pill and progesterone-only contraceptives, such as the contraceptive injection Depo-Provera, should be avoided as they can trigger or worsen existing acne. Some women report that their contraceptive pill has given them acne so discuss any skin changes with your doctor or nurse during usual pill checks.

Co-cyprindiol (POM)

Co-cyprindiol is a contraceptive pill that contains a medium dose of oestrogen, but also a drug called cyproterone acetate that combats the effects of testosterone in the body. It is marketed as Dianette® and is often prescribed for women who have acne and other signs of excessive testosterone such as excessive hair or obesity.

It is not uncommon to see a flare-up of the acne in the early stages of taking this treatment. However, it may take longer than the usual guidance of two months to start to see an improvement, so persevere before giving up. For some women, it may take up to four months to see the full benefit.

Although this treatment can make a significant improvement, it is prescribed only until the acne clears. Like the majority of other acne treatments, this one does not 'cure' the acne; it simply masks it, although it can do so very well. Coming off it just when the skin can look so good does seem illogical. Speak to your doctor or nurse if this worries you.

While this treatment can work well for some women, it can have the opposite effect for others. Like many other contraceptives, it may also give rise to mood swings, unwanted weight gain, headaches or more serious risks such as blood clots and heart problems. Be aware that coming off this treatment can result in the acne returning, as bad as it was before treatment started, so it is advisable to discuss using a topical treatment as a crossover which will help reduce any acne flare-ups.

If you require contraception at the same time as being prescribed this treatment, inform the person who has prescribed it for you and it can be prescribed free in England. As with all other contraceptive pills, be especially aware if you experience any dull throbbing pains in the chest or leg. Take any unusual pain seriously and report it to your doctor or practice nurse immediately.

CASE STUDY – ANDREA

I found the pill Dianette really fantastic, although it took a long time to 'kick in'. I almost gave up on it but then started to see my skin improve so dramatically that I stuck with it and felt like a new woman – I kept raving about my miracle cure and was recommending it to everyone I knew who had acne (even a boy wanted to know if he could try it!). But the bad news came when my GP told me I would have to come off it because I had been on it for longer than I was meant to (I had been on it for two years). I felt disappointed, but because my skin was so good, I thought I didn't need it any more anyway. I was so shocked when, within just three weeks, my skin got noticeably worse. It was just awful looking at my acne return. Within about two months it was like I had never taken the treatment at all. I was devastated. I went back to my doctor in tears and begged her to put me back on it. Luckily she agreed, after we discussed all the risks of going back on it again and for taking it longer than recommended. That was over two years ago now and I am frightened she will take me off it again. We talked about it last time I went to see her and she has suggested that I take a course of antibiotics whilst I come off the pill to help protect the skin from another acne flare-up. I will have to come off it eventually, so this sounds like good advice.

Isotretinoin (Roaccutane)

This is a controversial acne treatment that is considered, by some, to be a very powerful last-line option. Newspapers have both hailed its miracle benefits and condemned its reputed nasty side-effects. This section will take a look at the facts behind the headlines and allow you to draw your own conclusions.

Who it's for

Under tight European guidelines this drug, based on a synthetic form of vitamin A, can be prescribed only under the supervision of a dermatologist. UK guidance on when this tablet can be prescribed is quite clear and patients suitable for it should fulfil the following criteria:

1. Not responded to at least two courses of antibiotics
2. The presence of nodulo-cystic acne (the type most likely to scar)
3. Evidence of acne scars
4. Be psychologically distressed

How it works

Isotretinoin targets the sebaceous glands and, in effect, shrinks them. This also has an effect upon the oil production itself. The skin, soon after starting treatment, begins to have reduced levels of oil, which will often result in it becoming excessively dry. This dryness will often become more obvious through the course of treatment. Ironically, it may require the use of emollients usually reserved for eczema skin to help maintain a normal balance.

Although the main way it works is by targeting the oil glands, it also works on the skin cells, affecting how they are shed and reducing their blocking action within the hair follicle. As a result of these two effects, the main attraction for the bacteria on the skin is wiped out. The bacteria have nowhere to multiply so the redness, inflammation and pus-filled spots disappear.

A usual course of isotretinoin will last between four and six months, depending on how well the skin responds. One course alone is often enough, and while repeat courses can be given, the skin is usually so improved it is not necessary. For some, it may be likely they will need to use acne medication in the future, but the acne is usually less severe and easier to manage.

Side-effects

While the side-effects listed below are not the only ones, they are considered the most common. The chances of getting one or more from the list below are high, unlike with many other medicines. Anticipating these and taking steps to ensure they are either counteracted or carefully managed can help a person maintain a sense of control over their skin as well as the side-effects. The main side-effects are:

○ Dryness of the nose, eyes and lips. Sometimes the skin may become cracked and very dry, which may lead to bleeding in these areas
○ Headaches
○ Hair thinning (reversible)
○ Muscle aches and pains
○ Sensitivity to sunlight
○ Serious risks of abnormalities to an unborn baby, including death of the foetus

Managing side-effects

Acne flare-ups: It is usual to experience a flare-up of acne anywhere between 10 days and 6 weeks into taking isotretinoin. This can be very distressing for a lot of patients; however, if it is expected then it is less likely to result in feelings of despondency. If any flare-up persists beyond this period, or if the acne worsens rather than improves overall, then speak to your dermatologist or dermatology nurse about it. For some people a short course of steroids may be given to help reduce a flare-up, or the dose may be adjusted to help reduce side-effects.

Danger in pregnancy: All women of child-bearing age will be given careful counselling by a dermatologist or assigned to a specialist dermatology nurse who will support them during the course of medication. Women must be aware that the drug is incredibly dangerous to unborn babies, and taking it at the same time as pregnancy will often result in abnormalities or miscarriage. This can happen with taking even one single isotretinoin tablet, so its dangers cannot be overstated. Despite careful contraceptive planning and monthly pregnancy tests that must be carried out during the full course of treatment, some women have still fallen pregnant. This treatment does not have affect on future fertility and it is generally considered safe to try for a baby three months after completing a course, so anyone wishing for a baby needn't feel this treatment isn't for them. The monthly pregnancy tests taken under the supervision of either the dermatologist or dermatology nurse are time consuming but serve as a reminder of how important avoiding pregnancy is during treatment.

Dryness: Dryness of the eyes, nose and lips is very common. To help prepare for this, buy plenty of lip balm (any type will do) and make sure that there is enough to allow for everyday life. For example, put one in the car, in your handbag, in school bags and jackets, by the bed or next to the computer to be able to grab in an instant. Applying plenty of lip balm will help reduce extreme drying and cracked lips, which may lead to bleeding. Lip balm, or simple petroleum jelly (Vaseline®), can also be used in the nose to keep it moist. Artificial eye drops can help keep the eyes from over-drying. Some doctors recommend avoiding the use of contact lenses during this time, so make sure you have an up-to-date prescription pair of glasses ready to wear if needed.

Sun sensitivity: Reducing the chances of sensitivity to sunlight can be helped by applying plenty of oil-free sunscreen, ideally a minimum of factor 30, whatever the weather. This should be used every day during the course of treatment and applied regularly as directed (see page 208 and Chapter 12).

Waxing and exfoliating: Oral isotretinoin makes the skin more fragile and liable to scar. Plucking of hair and waxing should be avoided completely during the course and for one month afterwards.

Muscle aches and pains: Muscle aches and pains are more common in those who are highly active. If you are a keen sportsman or woman, tell the doctor when isotretinoin is prescribed and be prepared to experience some muscle aches and pains. If your sport is seasonal, such as football, discuss starting a course of isotretinoin at the end of the season to reduce the amount of exercise and physical stress the body undertakes during this period.

ISOTRETINOIN AND DEPRESSION

Much of the publicity surrounding this treatment also includes concerns about depression. All UK dermatologists are well aware of this potential side-effect and should always counsel patients before starting a course. In a few cases where depression has been reported as a side-effect, some people have taken their own lives or been deeply affected by a sudden onset of depressive symptoms where they felt bad enough to want to take their own life. It is not really possible to tell who might feel like this on a course, and certainly many patients report no such side-effect at all. One study at Boston University in 2000 questioned 20,000 acne patients. Some were using isotretinoin for their acne, others antibiotics. The team of scientists compared the risk of depression between the two groups and found that it was comparable in both.

However, in cases where patients report experiencing depressive symptoms while taking isotretinoin, there seems to be a slightly increased risk of suicidal feelings occurring in those who have had a previous episode of depression before taking isotretinoin. Also, some patients have reported feelings of anxiety or agressive behaviour. For this reason, the treatment should be used with caution in these people and only after careful consideration of all the risks and benefits.

Any serious changes in mood may be difficult to notice when it happens to you; being able to get an outside perception will be very helpful, especially if the changes are gradual. It might help to enlist someone you trust before starting a course of isotretinoin to be your 'mood gauge'; ask them to share an honest opinion on any signs of changes that may indicate depression. These changes may be subtle or obvious (or completely absent of course), but it has given many worried parents, friends and patients a degree of reassurance to know there is someone looking out for them in this way. As part of this agreement you may wish to discuss what to do should you show such signs, and draw up your own 'depression action plan' to decide in advance about anything you will want to do, even if that means having to withdraw from treatment. All this can be discussed both with your chosen person and your doctor or nurse who has prescribed the treatment.

Is isotretinoin the right treatment for me?

This is up to each individual. A decision on whether to take it or not should depend upon full discussion with a dermatologist and consideration of whether the benefits are believed to outweigh the risks sufficiently. If a person who is offered this treatment has one of the type of acnes described on page 23, and if they are fully aware of the side-effects and how to manage them, then weighing up the pros and cons might be straightforward. Nobody should tell another person whether they think it is right for them; this includes doctors and nurses, some of whom have reportedly scared patients because they are ignorant of the drug's benefits and focus only on the risks. A decision to take it should be based firstly upon medical opinion. If the doctor prescribing it is satisfied that the treatment is appropriate for the type of acne, then each patient must decide for themselves. Sometimes it may not feel right, or the patient may feel very anxious about taking it. In these circumstances it might be sensible to try alternative prescribed acne medication and defer a decision about isotretinoin to another time.

Some helpful questions to ask yourself may include:

○ Am I satisfied that I have given other treatments a good enough chance to really work? Did I take or use them as I should have done?
○ Is my skin scarring?
○ Am I so unhappy with how I look that it is affecting my self-esteem?
○ Do I understand the benefits against the risks?
○ Have I put the right questions to the right people?
○ Should I try something else first?
○ What other options might I have?
○ Am I prepared to put up with the side-effects?

Isotretinoin cannot be guaranteed to work for everybody, but it is still considered a gold standard treatment for hard-to-treat, scarring acne. While it may not give a permanent solution, it can help to knock the acne switch down a notch or two by reducing the size of the oil-producing glands. Some doctors have reported that between 30 and 50 per cent of people taking a course of isotretinoin find that acne returns to some degree. However, further courses can be offered.

Taking a second or third course of isotretinoin

Some dermatologists see patients for a second, third or even fourth time following the initial course of this treatment. Taking more than one course is acceptable unless the first course gave rise to concerns about side-effects including depression. For some, their acne does return but not as aggressively as before, and a course of other prescribed treatment will be sufficient to keep it firmly under control. There will usually need to be a gap between courses to give the skin a chance to recover and to make a reassessment before a decision to re-prescribe is taken.

CASE STUDY – LOTTIE

My skin had been getting worse in my last couple of years at school. I was given the nickname 'Spotty Lotty', which seemed to stick and really got on my nerves. I was self-conscious about my skin and found myself making excuses not to go out when it was really bad. I remember one spot I had which was evil – it was literally on the end of my nose and not only was it huge, it was really, really painful. It was all I could see on the outside of my vision and for me it was the last straw.

I had tried loads of other things for my skin. Dianette worked really well but my family named me the 'nightmare child from hell' when I was on it and I had to come off it before my family disowned me! I think all my feelings about my skin came to a head with that last huge boil. I decided that I really had to sort it out so I would never have to look in a mirror and feel so repulsed again.

My doctor was really helpful and he referred me to the dermatologist who suggested I try Roaccutane. I had an appointment with the nurse who spent a long time with me going over everything I might need to know about it, and was asked to take a pregnancy test there and then so I could get started straight away. I didn't think it would happen that fast, but I felt I had been given enough time to ask my questions and to appreciate the importance of not getting pregnant. I decided that I would abstain from sex during my treatment just to be sure – that's how important it was to me to clear my skin!

I had a couple of hitches during the course. Firstly my skin went so dry that I found it almost impossible to keep moist; then my lips dried so badly that they would bleed every morning – I felt like a smile was the biggest torture, so decided to give up smiling too (actually I learnt that I smiled more than I thought by having to do this!). I found a brilliant intensive-care lip balm and used loads of it – every day, every hour, every time I ate or drank anything – and it did help.

When I started university I had to move away. As I had been instructed to go to see the nurse each month and give a negative pregnancy test, this was going to be very difficult – my university was 275 miles away. Luckily, the dermatology nurse at the hospital, Julie, was brilliant and we made an arrangement with my university doctor that my results would be faxed to the dermatology unit in my home town; they would then issue the prescription which would be sent to me. This was the best solution, and although it was a pain for everyone it did work out well in the end.

That was five years ago and my skin is absolutely great now – it's what I would class as 'normal' and I feel like I have been liberated. My eyes are really itchy still, especially the skin around the eyes which never seems to be anything but dry, but being spot-free is great. I can live with the scarring, but I can't imagine not having taken the isotretinoin – the thought of still having skin like that is really depressing.

Treating Acne in Unusual Areas of the Body

Hairline acne (pomade acne)

When it first appears, acne is likely to follow the 'T' zone covering the forehead and down the nose where the grease glands are most highly concentrated. Areas where greasy hair comes into contact with the skin may cause acne breakouts.

If the acne appears around the hairline, then a few simple steps could help reduce the problem. Firstly, it is not realistic to expect someone who has acne in these areas to keep hair scraped back and off the face to show the world the spots, but it will be useful to keep contact with greasy hair and skin to a minimum. Therefore, wash hair as frequently as possible. If the skin underneath a fringe doesn't get much breathing space, use face wipes to remove surface grease during the day (any type of wipe will do, although antibacterial may be preferred). This helps to reduce blockages that will attract the spot-making bacteria. If you usually wear make-up, remove all traces every night.

If you use hair products that contain grease or anything likely to block the skin, such as pomades or gels, then keep contact with the skin to a minimum. Wipe away any excess hair products from the hairline area. Use acne products in this area, but be careful with benzoyl peroxide (see pages 56–7) as it is also a bleaching agent. If it touches the hair, it will bleach it, and this includes any facial hair such as beards and eyebrows!

'Backne' (acne on the back)

Acne on the back can be hard to treat because it is awkward to reach, so applying creams or washes to this area will be challenging. If you are being prescribed treatment for acne that also appears on the back, consider the following:

1. Ask the doctor to give you the largest size of any topical creams or lotions they intend to prescribe as they will need to go further.
2. If you would prefer not to struggle to put creams on yourself, or know that you don't have someone to help you, then ask the doctor for tablets instead.
3. Consider investing in a 'body baster', a simple tool made of plastic designed to spread creams onto the back area. It can be used to apply any products such as sun creams, fake tans, emollients or acne treatments. These are available online and at some pharmacists.

SELF-MEDICATION FOR 'BACKNE'

You can self-treat back acne just as you would acne on any other area of the body, but because of its location, scrubs and other recommended self-treatments may be harder to apply. You can try using your usual facial treatments on the chest and shoulders, which is best done in the shower. Use your towel to give a vigorous body rub to help exfoliate the skin. Back brushes might be worth trying to give an extra exfoliating effect. However, be careful not to knock the top off any spots on your back.

Despite the best medical advances in acne treatment, there will always be the challenge of being able to physically reach areas of the back. The best way to be sure to get the treatment onto the affected areas is to ask someone for help.

The broad range of treatment options should mean that no one has to put up with acne. However, finding the best treatment may take time and effort, which can be frustrating. As long as you stick to the guidelines in this chapter, you are likely to find a solution that works best for you. Remember to ask for help from your family doctor or nurse if you are at all worried about your skin.

Treating Acne with Lights and Lasers

When these types of treatment first appeared, they caused a sensation in the media. Many were hailed as 'miracle treatments' and alternative ways of getting rid of acne, safely and (relatively) painlessly. With over a decade passing since they were first introduced, the jury is still out. Some studies have given encouraging results, but some have failed to show a convincing effect. Patients have reported a preference for these therapies because they need to be used only once every few weeks, as opposed to everyday medications that may have side-effects.

Both lights and laser treatments used to help acne (and rosacea) operate on different wavelengths and work in different ways. Lasers have traditionally been used to resurface the skin by burning (ablating) to remove the layers at microscopic levels. These ablative laser may need to be used under general or local anaesthetic. The skin may take several weeks to heal as the new 'crust' or scab that forms afterwards needs to fall off, revealing new skin beneath (for more information, see 'Laser treatments', Chapter 6, pages 130–1). New lasers have been introduced especially to help acne. These avoid damaging the surface of the skin, and instead work in a non-ablative way. They can target either the sebaceous glands, the main culprit in acne, or the bacteria which feed on the oil.

Lights to treat acne

This type of technology uses a broad-spectrum light beam of either red or red and blue light combined, and their primary action is to kill the *P. acne* bacteria and promote healing. This type of light treatment is usually totally painless and can be used on an ongoing basis to help prevent acne.

Red and blue light technology is not the same as facial tanning units, which emit harmful UV rays. Instead the waves of light fall outside of the harmful light rays: with blue light at 415 nanometres and red at 660 nanometres.

This type of treatment can be purchased for home use in a convenient box which rests on a table top, although they are also available in some beauty salons. Examples include Britebox®, OmniluxTM and ClearLight®.

PROS AND CONS OF LIGHT THERAPY

Pros:
- The gadget has a wide appeal to boys
- Is painless to use
- Can be used in conjunction with most acne treatments, except isotretinoin or topical retinoids

Cons:
- Needs to be used daily
- Takes longer than usual acne treatments, up to 15 minutes a day
- Bulbs can be expensive to replace
- Eye protection must be used
- Can be expensive to purchase but cost-effective if used regularly

PROS AND CONS OF USING LASERS FOR ACNE

Pros:
○ Doesn't have lasting side-effects
○ Doesn't require daily (or twice daily) treatment, so nothing is needed between sessions
○ Can help improve the general tone and texture of the skin, reducing the appearance of scars

Cons:
○ Can be quite painful/uncomfortable
○ Requires time and effort to travel to clinics
○ Expensive compared with prescription options

Intense Pulse Light (IPL) is another type of light-based treatment for helping acne. It uses yellow and green light in addition to red light and is administered via a hand-held device, which is passed over the skin in short pulses of light. Usually a chilled gel or an iced roller device is used on the skin to prepare it before the treatment as the heat generated by the intense pulse feels extremely hot. This type of treatment is not suitable for people with dark skin, and all patients undergoing a course of IPL will need to avoid sunlight for at least two weeks.

Lasers to treat acne

Lasers work by heating the skin for a very short period of time using a laser beam burst which blasts the skin. There is currently a choice of different types of lasers, although one of the most established is the yellow light laser. This yellow light laser targets the prophorine, a substance found inside the *P. acnes*, and kills it by producing oxygen, which is the known enemy of this bacteria. Yellow light laser also has the benefit of boosting the formation of collagen (which helps to plump the skin), so it may have the added benefit of improving the appearance of scarring. Other lasers work closer to a near-infrared beam.

Doctors seem divided on the benefits of lasers to help acne and many studies seem to give conflicting results. It can be difficult to choose between the lasers as they are usually very expensive to purchase and each clinic will be inclined to promote its own in preference to others, so getting a non-biased opinion is very difficult. Examples of such lasers include the N Lite® and Smoothbeam®.

CASE STUDY – CRAIG

My mum kept nagging me to do something about my bad skin. She would moan that I hadn't washed properly, but she didn't really know how much my skin bothered me – my girlfriend had finished with me because I wouldn't go out when my skin was bad and I used to keep getting her to buy me stuff for my skin. I basically felt really fed up with it all and decided to check out the internet to have a look at what might be available that didn't involve slapping on bad-smelling creams and stuff that needed to be left on overnight.

I found a really interesting alternative that claimed to work by using light waves, and wouldn't need me to use other treatments. It looked like an old-fashioned mobile phone, covered in small blue lights. You hold it directly on your face for a few minutes and move it around the skin where you usually get spots. What I liked about it was that it was painless and really easy to use. It cost about the same as what I would spend in a year trying creams from the chemist, so I think that makes it worthwhile for me. It took a few weeks to get better but it was worth waiting because my skin seems to have improved overall now, so I can't recommend it enough. The one I use is called 'Acne Star', but there are lots more types available, some that use red and blue light and some that you sit in front of like a box people use for seasonal affective disorder. Having said how brilliant I found this, I recommended it to someone else at college who also had bad skin and they thought it was rubbish!

CHAPTER FOUR

ALTERNATIVE AND COMPLEMENTARY ACNE TREATMENTS

As well as the conventional acne treatments described in the last chapter, there are also alternative and complementary therapies available. While there is generally scant evidence for the effectiveness of such remedies, some people prefer to use them instead of conventional acne treatments, while others are willing to try both. 'Alternative' treatments are those used in place of conventional medicine, whereas 'complementary' therapies are used alongside it. The options available seem almost endless, from Indian remedies and Chinese herbs to aromatherapy and acupuncture. With such choice it can be difficult to know where to begin.

Medicines licensed for use in the UK need to go through a rigorous process of investigation for both safety and effectiveness. In other words: are they safe and do they do what they say they will? Other considerations may be the balance between the benefits of a product and the risks of unwanted side-effects. If a product has been carefully evaluated in this way, you can usually be reassured that what you are taking has a good degree of background data and a system for monitoring it on an ongoing basis. However, if a product hasn't gone through these tests it may not be possible to know exactly what you are taking, especially if it is purchased through the internet.

Buying Treatments Online

A word of caution. While the internet has provided the opportunity for millions to explore self-treatments, be aware of the potential pitfalls of purchasing in this way. Firstly, if purchasing from abroad, some goods may be subject to import tax, may be banned from being imported, and may also be counterfeit or poor quality copies of licensed drugs. It is illegal to obtain drugs in this way. Even UK websites may be selling counterfeit products. A site may appear to be professional, but claims such as 'No prescription required' and 'No questions' should make you question how trustworthy it is.

If a site is genuinely professional it will always:

○ give options for online advice
○ display an address/phone number (not just a PO box or a mobile number)
○ have a privacy and security policy/statement
○ be a member of a recognised professional organisation such as the Royal Pharmaceutical Society of Great Britain (RPSGB)

If it is an online pharmacy, it should offer access to a professionally qualified pharmacist or be run under the management of a qualified pharmacist. Always seek professional advice before considering purchasing online remedies, either conventional or alternative/complementary.

TOP TIPS FOR ALTERNATIVE/COMPLEMENTARY TREATMENTS

Some sensible questions to ask about any complementary or alternative treatment before trying it are:

○ What does this contain? (Some remedies may contain traces of nuts, for example.)

○ Is it possible I might react badly to this type of treatment, and if so, what should I do?

○ How long do I need to use it for before I notice any results? (If this is longer than two months then ask why.)

Beliefs about Complementary and Alternative Acne Treatments

When doctors train at medical school, they are taught to investigate science and apply scientific principles to their work. They seek to understand evidence and to use medicine that can be proved, through carefully constructed studies, to have benefit. It may not be reasonable, therefore, to expect GPs to share your beliefs about complementary or alternative treatments if the evidence for them is scarce or hard to find.

Doctors are also encouraged to adhere to NHS prescribing guidelines, which are reviewed carefully by government health watchdogs. Chinese, homeopathic and Indian medicines have not gone through the same scientific processes. If doctors are not working with such remedies on a regular basis, they are unlikely to understand much about them – either their pros or cons. They will not usually be able to make an informed statement on their likely benefit. It's not part of their job description. However, they will probably need to know if you are taking or using any type of complementary or alternative treatment listed in this section, as there may be some interaction between it and conventional medicines.

Medical doctors and alternative/complementary practitioners rarely share the same beliefs and come from different approaches and backgrounds. It may not be reasonable to expect an insightful and honest opinion from a practitioner of one type on the benefits (or otherwise) of what a practitioner of the other type does.

QUICK TIPS

○ Always tell your doctor or nurse about any complementary treatments you are taking or using as it may interfere with prescribed treatments.

○ Tell your complementary practitioner if you are on any prescribed treatments.

○ Avoid stopping any prescribed treatments without first getting advice from your doctor or nurse.

A holistic approach

Modern doctors and nurses are trained to look at symptoms and treat them with the aim of reducing diseases and illnesses. They do not usually need to take into account diet, lifestyle or general well-being, although this information may be useful to decide on which medicines or types of treatment to prescribe. However, alternative practitioners usually do the opposite; they believe that symptoms reflect what is going on inside a person and that it is not enough to treat the symptom on its own. They will seek to treat the 'whole person', which is a holistic approach. 'Holistic' originates from the

Greek word 'holism', meaning *all, entire, total*. This approach involves taking into account the whole of a person, including their physical, biological, emotional and mental needs.

In recent years there has been a push for doctors and nurses to take into account the 'whole' person. Treating holistically has significant meaning in areas of healthcare such as care of the dying and birthing plans for mums-to-be. However, many doctors and nurses do not have the time, resources, knowledge or enthusiasm for such approaches, which is why many patients come away from a rushed consultation feeling they have not been truly listened to.

The benefit of visiting an alternative or complementary practitioner may be that there is more time allowed to discover more about the patient. This would include sharing far more information than just a list of symptoms. However, this will often come at a price. Such practitioners work in the private sector, meaning their work is not subsidised by NHS funds. This can make them expensive to visit; treatment costs may run into the hundreds, or even thousands, of pounds. As well as the costs, some people worry that in some 'professions' there is a lack of regulation and standards in training, meaning that anyone with a bit of knowledge can set up a practice.

It is useful to note that many of the practices listed in this section have professional bodies. They regulate and register their members, who usually have to prove their experience. However, for some, this may still be only a minimal level. Always contact the regulating body or association for advice. Find a practitioner through such organisations rather than turning to local advertising. Ideally, ask friends for recommendations.

Is natural best?

Just because something is natural, does that make it safer or better? Using raw ingredients or products that come from plants, trees or seeds may fit into a person's beliefs that this is preferable to something processed and full of chemicals. It's true that many alternative/complementary therapies are based on ancient remedies that were used long before the introduction of chemical compounds and processes. However, that is not to say that some of these remedies may not be harmful to vulnerable groups and fatal reactions to herbal medicines sometimes occur. Children, people with weak immune systems, the elderly and pregnant or breastfeeding mothers should use such remedies with caution and only on medical advice. Some natural products, such as St John's Wort, which is commonly used for helping depression, give some people unwanted side-effects such as headaches, raised blood pressure, vomiting or sensitivity to sunlight. Many acne remedies may give other unwanted effects, such as dryness, peeling, stinging or burning, just as you might expect from prescription products. Any side-effects can usually be managed in the same way as for prescription treatments (see Chapter 3).

A to Z of Alternative and Complementary Therapies

While this list represents the main options, it doesn't necessarily include them all.

Acupressure (shiatsu)

Shiatsu literally means 'finger pressure'. It was used by Chinese monks over 5,000 years ago, since when it has developed into the therapy used today. Shiatsu is based on the same principles as acupuncture (see below) but without the needles, concentrating on meridians or energy lines. Everything is related to the five main elements that correspond to different parts of the body:

○ Fire – heart
○ Water – kidneys
○ Wood – liver
○ Earth – spleen
○ Metal – lungs

Like acupuncture, the aim of shiatsu is to seek balance in the life energy of the body. When the balance becomes disturbed we become unwell or develop diseases or conditions that affect certain parts of the body. Shiatsu uses a series of finger pressures all over the body, following the meridians or pathways. It claims to help rebalance the body's energies, regulate the function of the organs and improve circulation. It aids the body to self-heal by releasing its natural energy flow. Shiatsu practitioners will often use their elbows, feet or knees as well as their fingers during therapy, but they rarely use the palms of their hands.

Acupuncture

Acupuncture is thought to have originated over 2,500 years ago. It remained largely unknown outside Asia until the 1970s. Now it is recognised by the NHS as a valid treatment for back pain. The underlying belief is that health conditions, illnesses and pain occur when the body's *qi*, or vital energy, cannot flow freely. The body's energy meridians can become obstructed, like a trapped nerve or blocked pipe. This can happen for any number of reasons, such as stress, poor nutrition, infection or injury.

By inserting ultra-fine, sterile needles into specific acupuncture points, a traditional acupuncturist aims to re-establish the flow of *qi* to restore balance and generate the body's natural healing response. Traditional acupuncturists aim to treat the person as a whole rather than just the disease or condition. They also, like many other holistic practitioners, consider all lifestyle, emotional and environmental factors before beginning treatment.

Aromatherapy

This is the practice of using essential oils for therapeutic purposes. Aromatherapy appears to have been used since the first century, becoming more popular in recent times. Essential oils give their benefits through their aroma (healing scents) and by application to the skin. Oils are usually extracted either by steam distillation (such as eucalyptus oil) or by squeezing (such as grape seed oil). They may be used neat or by diluting in a carrier oil to allow application to the skin.

It is worth noting that carrier oils may worsen acne as they tend to block the skin in a similar way to oils produced by the sebaceous glands. Therefore, for treating acne problems there are two main oils with anti-microbial (antibiotic) effects that can be applied without diluting in carrier oils: tea tree oil and lavender oil. Research into tea tree oil has revealed that its benefits can be compared to those of benzoyl peroxide.[1] Use these oils sparingly and be aware that they can cause drying and flakiness. For a homemade moisturiser, add a drop of either oil to aloe vera gel (about 5 per cent oil to 95 per cent aloe vera).

CASE STUDY – CONNOR

I prefer to use natural products on my skin and wasn't happy using harsh creams like the benzoyl peroxide my chemist recommended. I certainly wouldn't want to use antibiotics of any type. I have a friend who is an aromatherapist and swears by the benefits of essential oils for all sorts of health problems, so it seemed a good idea to try it for my acne. I was advised to use tea tree oil and lavender oil twice a day. Although my acne was never severe, my spots have all but gone. If I do have a particularly bad breakout I will use neat tea tree oil on the individual spot – this beats those harsh products you buy in the chemist any day. It's using nature to help heal the skin and I swear by it.

Ayurvedic medicine

This word originates from two Sanskrit words meaning life and knowledge. Ayurvedic medicine can be traced back over 3,500 years and is said to have been passed down by Hindu gods. It is still the basis for medicines used throughout the Indian subcontinent. Treatments are a mixture of detoxifying, diet, exercises, herbs and a variety of techniques that target mental and emotional health. Its aims are to work with the body's natural forces rather than against them.

In Ayurveda, the tridosha – the three doshas or energetic forces in the form of tissues – control all activities of the body. The three doshas are:

○ Vata
○ Pitta
○ Kapha

In acne, kapha and vata are the two main doshas that cause problems. Massages and face packs may be part of an Ayurvedic treatment plan, as well as changes of lifestyle in order to help balance these three vital energy forces.

Chinese herbal medicine

This type of treatment consists of more than just taking medicines. It focuses on the body's Yin and Yang. These are two complementary principles, with Yin representing negative, dark and feminine qualities, and Yang the positive, bright and masculine. Chinese medicine aims to keep these balanced in order to maintain good health. Like many other complementary treatments, it will take into account a person's lifestyle, general health and other issues that may affect the body's normal functions. It will usually draw upon a variety of remedies including herbal medicines, teas, acupuncture (see above), dietary changes and breathing exercises.

Chinese herbal medicine claims to help acne problems by addressing the digestive system. This is thought to be weakened, resulting in excessive toxic substances in the body. Acne is also considered to be the result of increased cholesterol intake. Treatments will usually focus on the cholesterol as well as the digestive problems. Chinese herbalists believe that this imbalance is due to the overflow of Yang, which produces too much heat. To help restore balance, herbs that relieve the accumulation of heat and reduce toxins are chosen.

Access to Chinese medicines is expanding, with many shops opening in local high streets and shopping centres. A wide variety of treatment options can be recommended, although the teas are often reported to taste bitter and unpleasant and can rarely cause severe side effects (e.g. hepatitis).

Herbal medicine

This term describes a wide variety of medicines that originate mainly from plants or herbs, although this can also include honey, shells or animal parts. It may have started with earliest humans observing sick animals selecting plants to aid healing. While Chinese herbal medicine has grown in popularity (see above), it is not the only type available, with almost all non-industrialised societies across the world using their own combinations of plants.

Herbal medicines are often used to treat a person over a long period of time, as much to heal as to prevent diseases and reduce symptoms including pain.

For acne, there are many types of herbal remedies. These include evening primrose and blackcurrant, and teas made of nettles, camomile or lavender. As well as recommending herbs, teas or oils, herbalists will suggest an acne-friendly diet. Lifestyle and general health will also be taken into consideration.

Homeopathy

The theory behind homeopathy is 'treat like with like', using what contributes towards the problem to help the problem. Whatever remedy is used will be heavily diluted in a carrier liquid followed by vigorous succussing (shaking). It is believed that the more it is diluted, the more potent it will be, which seems to be opposite to conventional medical beliefs. Homeopathic remedies can be given in tablet, powder, liquid or gel form. You would begin by having a consultation to give an in-depth picture of your general health and wellbeing, followed by a prescription tailored to your needs.

Hypnotherapy

The word hypnotherapy has origins in the Greek word 'hypnos', meaning sleep. This therapy aims to put a person into a hypnotic state to help them, via a qualified hypnotherapist, to explore their unconscious mind. Hypnotherapy has its roots in the belief that the unconscious can influence the conscious, meaning our actions and behaviour. It is already widely known that some people with skin conditions become depressed, anxious or withdrawn. While in a hypnotic state, these feelings are explored, allowing the person to identify positive intentions and beliefs about themselves.

It is hard to find evidence that hypnotherapy works as a treatment for acne. However, some practitioners believe that the skin is like a screen upon which we project our inner feelings. If feelings are suppressed, it is suggested this leads to the eruption of acne, the 'emerging feelings that can't be contained'. With the help of a qualified hypnotherapist, the person can be encouraged to identify and deal with these feelings.

Naturopathy

Naturopathy encourages the body to heal itself using natural remedies in harmony with the body's own rhythms. Practitioners may use a variety of methods to treat the patient. The first consultation will usually be spent exploring, in great detail, the person's emotional and physical state, as well as taking a medical history. Naturopaths will focus on diet and allergies and may recommend a variety of supplements and vitamins or diet and lifestyle changes. Acne is often considered to be a type of 'skin diabetes', where the person is not metabolising sugar properly. Chromium picolinate supplements may be recommended, as these are reported to improve glucose intolerance.

Reflexology

Reflexology works with the *qi* or 'life force' in the same way as acupressure (see above), using the foot as the main focus of manipulation to help diagnose and aid problems around the body. The theory is that each part of the foot relates to different areas (or zones) of the body, although the hand can be used in a similar way. Gentle manipulation and massage helps a person feel relaxed and their body is claimed to be rebalanced. Its benefits in acne are not widely acknowledged.

Vitamins and other supplements

In a normal balanced diet, most of us will gain the nutrients we need for everyday health. Supplements are usually necessary only if the diet is restricted in some way. However, there are a few vitamins and other supplements that are considered more key in aiding acne. They should be taken within usual recommended daily allowance (RDA) guidelines as doses beyond these may have a negative effect.

Omega 3 and Omega 6 essential fatty acids

These two essential fatty acids are commonly found in everyday diets. While both are necessary as the body cannot manufacture them, scientists claim they compete for limited space within cells. On a very basic level, Omega 3 is considered the 'good' oil and Omega 6 the 'bad' oil. This is not really justified, as both are needed by the body. However, in people with acne problems, Omega 3 is particularly recommended to help promote healing, fight infection and improve cell function. It is also claimed that Omega 6 is actually found in the sebum we produce in acne.

Trying to get a balance between the two is therefore recommended, with an ideal ratio of one part Omega 3 to three parts Omega 6. This might sound easy until you realise that modern western diets are full of Omega 6. At present many people are getting one part of Omega 3 for every twenty parts of Omega 6. To reduce Omega 6, cut down on the following:

○ Biscuits, cakes, confectionery
○ Margarine
○ Mayonnaise
○ Fried foods
○ Peanut butter

Try increasing Omega 3 by eating:

○ Cod liver oil
○ Soya beans
○ Tofu
○ Flax seed
○ Kiwi fruit
○ Nuts – particularly walnuts, pecans and hazelnuts
○ Eggs from free-range chickens

Vitamin A

Vitamin A has a variety of roles in the body's systems, including our vision, immunity and bone and skin health. Also known as a retinoid, vitamin A is used in prescription creams and can be very effective for acne; another form of it makes up the drug isotretinoin. Taken as a supplement, however, it will not really have enough impact to make a huge difference; it is reportedly quite easy to reach the RDA of 0.6 mg for women and 0.7 mg for men through a normal diet. A deficiency in this vitamin can lead to blindness. Too much vitamin A, however, is toxic and affects the liver, leading to death if taken in high enough doses. Post-menopausal women are advised to limit their daily intake to a maximum of 1.5 mg as it could be harmful to bone density. It should not be taken by pregnant women.

Foods naturally rich in Vitamin A include:

○ Cheese
○ Eggs
○ Oily fish
○ Liver
○ Sweet potatoes
○ Carrots
○ Broccoli

Vitamin B5

Research from a doctor in Hong Kong revealed that vitamin B5 (pantothenic acid) may be useful for acne because of its reported effects on oil production. However, there is great controversy about this particular vitamin as, in order to be of any effect, it needs to be taken at a very high dose for a continuous period. The usual RDA for vitamin B5 in an adult is 10 mg, but for those wishing to use it for their acne, doses of up to 10 g are suggested.

While there have been reports of some significant successes with vitamin B5, there are also strong warnings. For example, it might be the cause of other long-term health problems such as hair loss or ME (chronic fatigue). It is also recommended that other B-group vitamins are taken at the same time to avoid them being 'knocked out' by high B5 doses.

Foods naturally high in vitamin B5 include:

- Beef
- Eggs
- Brewer's yeast
- Kidney
- Liver
- Mushrooms
- Royal jelly
- Whole-wheat cereals and flour

Vitamin E

This has been hailed as the ultimate vitamin to help the skin heal. It is sometimes recommended in liquid form to rub directly onto the skin to help acne scarring. However, be aware that this can actually make acne worse for some people as the oil can block pores. Some people have complained it smells very oily and leaves the skin shiny.

Investigators have proposed a direct link between blood levels of vitamin E and the incidence of acne, according to a report[2] in a dermatology publication. The aim of the study was to investigate the blood levels of vitamin E in 100 newly diagnosed, yet untreated acne patients to establish if they had the same levels as 100 age-matched, healthy volunteers without acne. Overall, the healthy, acne-free group had higher amounts of vitamin E in their circulatory system than those with acne. Based on these findings, investigators concluded that low vitamin E blood levels could cause or aggravate an acne outbreak.

The RDA for vitamin E is 30 International Units (IU). While it can be found in many foods, this vitamin is often at low levels. Foods rich in vitamin E include:

- Almonds
- Wheat germ oil
- Sunflower seed kernels
- Sunflower oil
- Hazelnuts

The maximum level of vitamin E is 1,500 IU per day for adults, which can come from a combination of foods and supplements. Ideally, seek natural vitamin E supplements that are labelled 'D' (alternatively the synthetic form is labelled 'D, L').

Zinc

Applying zinc to the skin as part of an antibiotic/zinc combination can be very useful in managing acne (see page 66). Likewise, there are suggestions that zinc supplements can be helpful. It is believed zinc has anti-inflammatory properties with some small studies[3] showing an overall reduction in spots. However, the reason it works is a bit of a mystery, and zinc doesn't seem to help everyone.

Taking a zinc supplement over an extended period should be balanced with taking a copper supplement – the two will compete for absorption in the body and excess zinc will reduce absorption of copper. Becoming deficient in copper can affect energy levels, general wellbeing and hair growth. The daily recommended allowance for zinc is 5.5 to 9.5 mg for men and 4 to 7 mg for women. Current health recommendations advise against taking more than 25 mg zinc tablets a day.

Natural sources of zinc can be found in many foods, particularly proteins, including:

○ Meat
○ Milk
○ Dairy foods
○ Shellfish
○ Cereal products such as wheat bran

Vegetarians may get less zinc in their diets. They should eat plenty of dairy products such as milk and cheese, yeast, peanuts, beans, wholegrain cereals, brown rice, whole-wheat bread and seeds. Pumpkin seeds are thought to be one of the richest sources of zinc.

It seems ironic that many foods described as being rich in zinc are also singled out as potentially causing acne problems. According to some press reports, milk and other dairy foods are 'acne-genic' (likely to cause acne), but a closer look at details of the trials reveals many flaws. Apply the golden 'Two-Month rule' (see pages 46–7) before deciding if zinc is of benefit for your skin or not.

Changes to Diet and Lifestyle

Treating acne by focusing on diet and lifestyle considers the whole person, not just their skin. This approach suits some people's beliefs and values, and can be a helpful step towards solving acne naturally. Others may be more sceptical, perhaps finding that adjustments to their life take a lot of time and effort. For example, avoiding certain food groups altogether may be hard to fit in if you are a busy teenager on the go, or a mum trying to cook family meals. Whatever your beliefs, if you wish to try a change in diet it will undoubtedly take a lot of effort. These tips may help:

○ Keep a food and skin diary: record what you eat every day and the condition of your skin. This will enable you to see if your skin changed in any way while you were eating or avoiding certain foods.

○ Stick to any dietary changes for at least two weeks. Significant changes may take some time to be seen.

○ If you plan to change more than one food group, try it one group at a time. This will enable you to pinpoint which food group was responsible for changes in your skin.

Traditionally, any recommendations for changes in lifestyle will include not only diet, but sleep and stress factors too, as these can be the culprits in many health problems. It is, however, easier to say you need to get more sleep and to relax than to actually achieve it! If you are serious about making changes to your life to help you feel less stressed then consider the following:

○ Be sure you understand what type of changes you need to make to your life. Being told to relax more doesn't describe how it should be done. How do you plan to relax? What makes one person relax may cause another person to fall asleep with boredom!

○ Introduce any lifestyle change gradually, rather than making huge changes overnight. This gives you a chance to get used to it, whether it involves taking 10 minutes out of every day to meditate or joining a dance class. Enjoy the achievements of every small change rather than expecting overnight changes. Ironically, drastic changes may be stressful because they put you under too much pressure.

○ Avoid making a change in lifestyle and diet a New Year resolution. Statistics suggest that just over 50 per cent of people who make these resolutions believe they can be achieved but only 12 per cent actually do so! You don't want to set yourself up to fail.

Although there is a lack of strong evidence to prove that diet and lifestyle changes make a huge difference to the skin, there are many cases to support the theory that these types of change have a positive impact. It is important to appreciate the feel-good factor of adopting positive lifestyle changes that focus on relaxation and a healthy balanced diet. That is something which, ultimately, we would all benefit from, no matter what the condition of our skin.

CHAPTER FIVE
EMERGENCY SPOT SOLUTIONS

Sometimes a spot appears at the time it is least wanted; maybe just before a first date or a day before a wedding or special event. The skin seems to have the knack of knowing when it is most important to look its best and then doing everything it can to ignore it! Don't despair, because although prevention is better than cure, some options can help in emergency situations. Bear in mind, though, that it is also possible to make the skin look far worse, so be careful. Only touch the skin or use emergency spot products if you have an outbreak that will affect you in some negative way. The best advice is to leave the skin alone whenever possible.

This chapter does not attempt to belittle or undervalue the importance of treating acne properly, as outlined in Chapters 3 and 4. It merely acknowledges that up to 95 per cent of people with acne confess to having squeezed their spots.[1]

Squeezing Spots

It is human nature to want to squeeze your spots but doing so can make you feel guilty as it goes against most advice. When you look in the mirror and see an even redder face or bleeding spots, you might wish you hadn't given in to temptation. The following tips will help you decide whether it is a good idea to proceed with squeezing spots and, if so, how to go about it.

Knowing when to start

We all have different ideas about what sort of spots need to be touched and which should be left alone. Before deciding to touch any spots think:

○ Is this spot ready? (see guide below)
○ Am I due to face other people and, if so, can I definitely *not* leave this spot alone?
○ Is it at least four hours before I need to go out or meet others?
○ Am I prepared to risk making it look worse?

If you answer 'yes' to more than three of the above, then go for it. However, *only* proceed using the guide below.

Knowing when to stop

Like any secret habit or indulgence, when it comes to squeezing spots it is always advisable to stick to moderation rather than going over the top. This advice is especially true if you find yourself continually picking the skin or examining it in minute detail using a mirror under harsh lighting. This behaviour has been linked to obsessive compulsive disorder (OCD) which may also include behaviours such as hand washing, hair pulling or the need to check light switches are off and so on. Follow these tips:

○ Stick to the 'traffic light guide' rules (see below) and avoid returning to spots that have recently been squeezed.

○ Clear liquid in a squeezed spot is a sign that the spot has been squeezed too hard or for too long so avoid this whenever possible.

○ Set a timer if necessary and allow yourself no more than five minutes in front of the mirror. Just walk away if after this time you have still not managed to clear the spots you hoped to.

TRAFFIC LIGHT GUIDE TO SQUEEZING SPOTS

This is probably the most simple and easy-to-remember guide ever! There are, however, a few basic rules to consider first:

○ Once you have squeezed a spot, leave it alone.

○ Use only freshly washed hands or a clean tissue.

○ Avoid digging long nails into the skin. This not only damages the skin but also leaves large marks behind.

○ Use a concealer only once the skin has started to settle (this may take up to an hour).

○ You can use emergency spot treatments to help calm and reduce redness.

THE GUIDE

Think traffic lights:

Red – stop! Squeezing red spots (papules) hard may force the contents deeper in to the skin. This can cause greater damage, possibly resulting in a scar which might not have happened had the spot been left. A papule can be treated with emergency spot products that help to reduce the redness, and can then be concealed with a product that matches the usual skin colour. This is suitable for both men and women.

Yellow – ready! This type of common spot, called a pustule, has a yellowish centre filled with pus. Pus is the name given to the white blood cells that are fighting the bacteria causing the spot. This can be gently squeezed out using the following technique to keep any damage to the skin to a minimum:

○ First use a warmed face cloth and leave on the spot for a few minutes to help prepare the area to make it easier to squeeze.

○ Gently pull the skin apart around the spot, away from the centre. It is natural to want to squeeze together, but this can make the spot worse. If it is ready, the action of pulling apart should be enough to allow it to gently pop. Any more pressure could lead to problems.

○ If you have to use long or sharp nails, wrap two pieces of clean tissue around your fingers to give plenty of padding.

○ Avoid the temptation to pierce the skin, and don't use home-sterilised pins or needles.

○ Stop if you see blood, carefully dab at the skin and leave alone to recover.

○ Dab the skin after it has burst and apply any self-medication that claims to help calm redness.

○ Leave the skin as long as possible before trying to conceal.

○ If all of the above don't work, leave the spot alone.

In case you are wondering about the last colour of the traffic light, if you have a green spot, you will need to seek help from your doctor! Luckily this is extremely rare and not usually connected to acne in any way.

CASE STUDY – CARRIE

I heard about the 'traffic light guide' and it really made me chuckle because at first it didn't make a lot of sense (I was thinking in particular about green spots!). However, once I realised the theory behind it – you can only go near a spot that is not red – it made perfect sense. As someone who has been a compulsive skin picker for a number of years, I have noticed how my skin looks very blotchy underneath my foundation. I have never been able to leave my skin alone, and this guide sort of gives me permission to have a go, yet know when to stop. I think it's good to acknowledge that we are all human and everyone has a go at squeezing their zits from time to time. In my case, though, I would get a bit carried away; that was until I heard about the guide. Now I don't feel quite so compulsive and hear myself saying, 'Okay, that's where you stop now, especially when my timer pings after 5 minutes!'

Emergency Spot Treatments

Some old wives' tales may have an element of truth in them when it comes to what can help spots in the short term.

Toothpaste

There is still no evidence to support the use of this, yet many people claim it helps to calm the redness of a spot (it is also used for the same reason to conceal 'lovebites'). One theory behind its varying success is that it contains triclosan, an ingredient found not only in toothpaste but also some skin, shaving and household cleaning products. Its antibacterial properties may help to reduce the redness of a spot, but a white lump of toothpaste on your face will look far more obvious! Another theory about toothpaste is that it acts as a type of mop to help absorb and draw out a spot. However, it can also leave the skin looking bright red – so be aware!

Clay-based face masks

The effect of drawing out or absorbing the contents of a spot can also be achieved by using a clay-based face pack. If you don't have

REMOVING BLACKHEADS

Blackheads, or open comedones, are usually black and can be straightforward to extract by following the same method recommended for squeezing spots. They will usually require a little extra pressure behind them after pulling apart, and it may be necessary to follow this by gently squeezing inwards to help the comedone clear up. They will usually leave a tiny hole while the skin takes a day or two to recover.

Some gadgets have been invented that help to remove blackheads without having to physically squeeze with fingers, but they basically do the same job. One such option is a comedone 'spoon'. This small metal ring on a stick is pressed against the skin while keeping the comedone in the centre. Pushing against the skin should, in theory, release the contents. However, this can leave an extra ring mark against the skin, making it look more obvious.

The other choice is an adhesive strip. This uses a type of glue to stick to the skin. When removed, it extracts the contents of the comedones. Feedback on this method is generally positive and it is not reported to damage the skin.

time to apply one to the whole face, dab on to the affected area and leave on for as long as possible (up to the recommended time). This can be helpful if you have just squeezed a spot and need to dry it out quickly. Rinse, pat dry and leave the affected area of skin until the last minute before applying any make-up.

Crushed aspirin

Aspirin is the same ingredient found in many face washes but is called by its chemical name, salicylic acid. Try crushing an aspirin (not paracetamol!) into a fine powder, adding a drop of water and applying the paste directly to the spot. Aspirin is not recommended for people aged under 16 or pregnant or breastfeeding women.

Ice

Ice's ability to numb and soothe skin might help calm any redness from a spot. Press a cube onto the skin for a few minutes.

CHAPTER SIX
ACNE SCARS AND MARKS: PREVENTION AND TREATMENT

Acne is one of the few dermatological conditions that cause scarring and long-lasting marks. As it is most likely to affect the face, it can leave a highly visible reminder of past acne. The good news is that not everybody will get scars and marks, and using the correct treatments as soon as acne appears will help prevent them.

Acne scars and marks can occur in any place affected by spots, including the back, chest and shoulders, and treating scars and marks in these parts of the body presents huge challenges. To make things worse, some scarring seems to get progressively more visible as the body ages because the skin's natural elasticity decreases and collagen is lost. Once past the age of 40, we can lose up to 1 per cent of our collagen each year, making our skin more prone to sagginess.

It is possible to avoid scarring and marking by following the good advice in this guide. Minimising the effects of existing scars and marks can also be achieved by an ever-widening choice of treatment options. Treating scars and marks, just like treating acne, will often demand patience and may not give 100 per cent improvement, so try to keep your expectations realistic.

Preventing Scars

Avoiding scars is a challenge, especially if the acne is severe or you develop deeper cysts. Common-sense steps to avoid or minimise the risks of scarring are:

○ Avoid picking or squeezing spots. If you do decide to squeeze a spot, follow the 'traffic light guide' in Chapter 5 (see pages 111–12). Only touch those spots that are ready to be squeezed, and never use force to burst the contents. Pushing, squeezing or pinching the skin hard can cause it to become damaged and inflamed, which may increase the chances of getting a scar.

○ Always use treatments as prescribed. Slapping on creams or doubling up tablets will not make the spots disappear more quickly; nor, more importantly, will it stop new spots forming.

○ Use the right type of treatment for the right type of spots (see Chapters 3 and 4).

○ Treat acne as soon as you get it – waiting too long will increase the chances of getting scars. You don't need to wait before you take action – choose from a range of medicated skincare products available in pharmacies or supermarkets and keep using them.

○ Don't wait – if you are worried that your skin is starting to scar, ask your doctor for help.

While some people end up with scarring, others may find their skin doesn't scar or mark at all. Whatever type of skin you have, it is important to take early action against spots. Stick to your treatments and, at the first signs of scarring, ask for a referral to a dermatologist.

Why do some people scar and not others?
It might be thought that scarring is a sign of a failure to treat acne effectively. However, this may be an unreasonable assumption as there are many other factors to take into consideration. These can include:

○ Being predisposed to developing scars. This can run in families, and some people who develop acne scarring have inherited their parents' skin types.
○ How severe the acne was, not necessarily how long the acne lasted.
○ Whether the skin was excessively picked or squeezed (not following the 'traffic light guide' to squeezing discussed on pages 111–12).

Different Types of Acne Scars and Marks

A scar is the result of damage to the skin. Each scar will appear different, even on the same person. There are various types of scar, although it is possible to be predisposed more to one type than another, and scars may be more severe in some areas than others. Scarring can either be seen as:

○ A change in pigment (although strictly speaking this is a mark, not a scar)
○ Raised above the normal level of the surface (hyper-trophic)
○ Pitted or dipped below the surface (atrophic)
○ Rolling scars (wave-like in appearance)

SKIN TYPES

Understanding what type of skin you have can help to ensure you keep your skin well protected from sun exposure, as well as helping you to choose the types of skin camouflage you might need.

FITZPATRICK SCALE OF SKIN TYPES

Type 1   Always burns, never tans; sensitive to exposure; redheaded, freckles

Type 2   Burns easily, tans minimally; fair-skinned, blue, green or grey eyes

Type 3   Burns moderately, tans gradually to light brown

Type 4   Burns minimally, always tans well to moderately brown; olive skin

Type 5   Rarely burns, tans profusely to dark; brown skin

Type 6   Rarely burns, least sensitive; deeply pigmented skin

Pigment changes

These marks are where the skin either loses the colour-giving cells known as melanocytes due to deep tissue damage from the spot or cyst, or produces more melanocytes. This is more commonly seen on the back. In the case of hypo-pigmentation (hypo meaning 'less'), the skin appears lighter, having little or no natural pigment. For others, especially in darker and Asian skin types, the damage left by a spot leaves a mark known as hyper-pigmentation (hyper meaning 'more'). In either case the skin is likely to recover over time but may not always return to the original colour. Although they may be very distressing, these flat marks can be quite easy to disguise using camouflage or concealers.

Hypertrophic (raised) scars

These scars rise above the surface of the skin but not beyond the area of the original spot. Many hypertrophic scars will settle eventually, leaving little or no scarring. However, if the scar grows beyond this area, it is known as a keloid scar (see below). Both of these types can be treated in the same way, although keloids tend to spread and be harder to control because they often return.

Keloid scars

A common type of hypertrophic scar is called 'keloid' scarring. This scar is more likely than normal hypertrophic scars to spread beyond the original area of 'injury' They occur when the skin lays down extra layers as a response to injury. These may look like little more than bumps, while some experience the skin 'bubbling' and growing around the area to huge proportions. Keloids happen because someone will be predisposed to getting them. They can result from any injury, not just acne – sometimes something as small as a scratch or bite (there have been cases where the original injury to the skin cannot be identified at all). Keloid scarring is formed of collagen, the natural fibre that maintains the skin's shape and texture. This overgrowth may appear shiny and be rubbery to touch but can also be quite painful or itchy. These scars seem to be more common in African and Asian skin types (skin type 6 on the Fitzpatrick scale, see page 119).

Atrophic (dipped) scars

This scarring is quite common in people who have acne and may appear in a few different varieties. These scars occur when the skin has lost collagen beneath the surface, like a soufflé that has collapsed, leaving a mini-crater similar to a saucer shape. Atrophic scars can be successfully treated for many people using a variety of techniques that aim to 're-plump' the skin and push the scar back to the same level as surrounding skin tissue.

Ice-pick scars

These dipped scars are the classic acne scars. Usually quite fine, they make the skin appear as if it has been punctured with an ice pick, hence the name. Because of their depth, it may be difficult to get good results from some types of laser or dermabrasion treatments (see pages 129–31), but some other options still remain.

Box-car scarring

This type of dipped scarring is angular and most commonly found on the temples and cheeks. It is similar to chickenpox scarring. These scars may look like they have been 'pressed' into the skin, similar to the impression that might be left after using a punch excision (when a tiny patch of skin is removed to be investigated). Where they differ to ice pick scars is that their edges are not sloped but vertical.

Rolling scars

These look wave-like as the name suggests. They happen because tissue beneath the top level of skin has become connected in fibrous bands, causing the skin to contract in places. This might be compared to rucks in a carpet when thread has been pulled underneath, leaving small ripples. In order to help these types of scar, they need to be released from underneath rather than from the top, similar to releasing the threads from beneath the snagging in the carpet.

Scar and Mark Treatments

Before you consider any treatment options, it might be helpful to think about your expectations. Each scar or mark will be different to the next. Sometimes one person may have every type of scar or mark described in this section; some of these may be deeper, older, newer, softer or harder than the ones next to it. No *one* particular treatment for scarring or marking will give a guaranteed improvement, despite some claims to the contrary. Scar tissue is a sign of damage to the skin, and treating that damage will usually require the skin to undergo more trauma, either by creams that 'dissolve' the top layers, or by a variety of other means. Skin that is delicate or scars easily may not respond so well to scar treatments.

Things to consider

A few key points to think about before considering any treatments for scars might be:

○ How do I feel about my scars? If you feel depressed about them, consider seeking advice about how you feel before undergoing invasive surgery. The treatments may not end up making you feel better at all.

○ How old is my scar? Give your skin plenty of time to settle down after acne. A recent scar is often only a sign of the skin healing (see below).

○ How much do I have to spend, or am I prepared to spend? Some scar treatments can be very expensive. The decision about how much you are willing to spend should depend upon what you need and what type of results you expect to achieve. Some companies offer credit and repayment options.

○ What if I am promised only a 30–50 per cent improvement? Will that be enough?

It may be helpful to consider these questions carefully before proceeding with scarring treatment options, especially those that carry more risk. There is the possibility that some might not work at all or leave the skin looking worse than before. Luckily this is rare, but make sure you get professional advice from someone you feel you can trust.

How old are the scars or marks?

Young scarring may heal naturally after a year, so try to leave new scars alone for as long as possible to give them a chance to improve on their own. Healing spots are also known as macules, and the red marks associated with them will usually fade away altogether. Try covering these with camouflage creams (see Chapter 11) or use a cosmetic concealer stick.

Where are the scars?

Acne is most likely to be seen on the face but it can also affect the neck, back, chest or shoulders. Having spots in these areas may also lead to scarring, especially as spots may be easily disturbed by clothing and body movement. This can, in turn, lead to the spot failing to heal properly, which can give an increased chance of scarring. This is why it is important to use treatments that help acne in these areas of the body and not just the face. There are also many challenges with scar treatment options on wider areas of the body:

1. Treating scars usually requires a 'grading in' system that graduates the edges to help blend in the break between the treated area and surrounding normal skin. This may

be difficult if the skin has widespread scars over a large area. The surgeon may be unwilling or unhappy to treat such scars because of the risk of infection following the procedure or because of the challenges of treating scars on a large body area. Patients may have difficulty with aftercare on areas such as the back because they are difficult to reach.

2. Scarring on the body, especially the back, may be difficult to reach to apply camouflage or other non-surgical procedures described later in this chapter.

3. The wider the body area to treat, the more expensive treatments will be.

Sun exposure

If you have had any type of ablative laser surgery or dermabrasion your skin will be more vulnerable to ultraviolet (UV) as the skin will be more damaged and may lose its natural pigment. It is vital to protect your skin from UV rays. You will need to wear a sun cream with a high protection factor throughout the year. If you are fair skinned, this change in skin colouring may not be too obvious, but the darker your skin tone, the more likely it is to be noticeable. If you are not willing to do this, then you may wish to think carefully before undergoing some of the more invasive options listed.

Skin type

It is unfortunate that the skin most likely to scar may also be the least likely to recover well from invasive procedures. If you are prone to getting raised scarring such as keloid scars (see page 120) then the procedures to help may also bring on a keloid scar. When considering your skin type, this includes the colouring of the skin.

Many of the options described in this chapter are invasive, meaning they dig below the surface, exposing skin that doesn't have the natural melanin which defines our colouring. If this is removed, the overall effect is to lighten the skin. If your skin type is 3 or higher on the Fitzpatrick scale (see box on page 119), then the removal of pigment will look very obvious.

It needn't feel like doom and gloom. There are still options for most people, including those with different skin colours and types as well as with deep or shallow scarring. New scarring will usually respond better to treatments than older scars, so once the acne has been successfully controlled, a sensible time to discuss treatments would be around six to twelve months from the last flare-up.

> If you have been treated with isotretinoin, you should leave any scar treatments for at least one to two months after treatment has stopped – you should consult your dermatologist or doctor. This is because the skin may be very delicate and will need time to recover.

Treating pigmentation marks

A small selection of off-the-shelf skincare products, such as oils and scar creams, claim to help reduce skin pigment changes that are commonly seen in pigmentation marks. Give them at least two months to see results before giving up. If they work, they will usually need to be used continuously to maintain improvement. Small trials of some of these products have claimed to show good results.

Some prescription creams that may help include azelaic acid, hydroquinone and topical retinoids. All these can reduce pigment changes but need to be used regularly for an ongoing period. They may have a bleaching effect on other areas of surrounding skin, so ask a pharmacist how to use them correctly before getting started. Any of these creams may leave the skin vulnerable to sun exposure, so it is advisable to use an acne-friendly sun cream at the same time. Ask your doctor or nurse about the benefits and risks of trying these treatments.

While treating pigmented marks, consider trying a concealer (equally suitable for men) or getting expert advice on skin camouflage, both of which can be used at the same time (see Chapter 11).

Treating keloid and hypertrophic scarring

There are choices for treating these scars, but none can give a 100 per cent guarantee to work. Unfortunately, some treatments designed to remove keloids may actually encourage more growth in the same area, especially if they have been surgically removed. However, many more can help. The options include one or more of the following:

Steroid injections

These injections are made directly into the tissue of keloid scars and are considered to be the most effective treatment. Their success is not always certain and they can be very painful, although local anaesthetic creams may be used. These injections will need to be given by a dermatologist. It might be difficult to find someone experienced in using this technique, so ask around before you commit to a course of treatment. To help speed the healing a special steroid-impregnated tape (Haelan® tape) can be applied.

Surgery

Surgery options may be available depending on the severity of the keloid, but there are still risks that the keloid may return. You will need a referral to your dermatologist or surgeon for further advice.

Cryosurgery

This involves freezing the scars but will also remove skin pigment so may not be suitable for skin types 3–6. This technique might be useful in conjunction with a course of steroid injections (see page 126).

Invisible gel sheets

These work on the same basis as pressure garments by applying pressure to the affected area. In effect, they compress the scar and help to prevent further growth. The sheets can be cut to size to fit around the scar and are transparent so can be used on any skin colouring. They need to be worn for up to 12 hours a day to get the best effect, and ideally as soon as the scar starts to appear. These are available from most pharmacists or on prescription. Skin camouflage (see Chapter 11) or daily make-up can be applied on top of gel sheeting.

Treating ice-pick and box-car scars

One way of working out how much improvement you might get from any treatment to an ice-pick scar is to gently stretch the skin apart. Whatever improvement you see by doing this is likely to be the degree of improvement you'll see after the treatment. As many ice-pick and box-car scars may be quite deep, home remedies or self-help products off the shelf may have little noticeable impact. Other options include the following:

Punch excision

The damaged area is removed using a punch excisor a bit like an apple corer, taking away a tiny round area that surrounds the damage. This new 'hole' over the old damage can then be neatly sewn or sutured (stuck) back together to make a new scar, which can be less noticeable than before. Steri-strips are used to help keep the skin together after this procedure, and some people advise keeping them on for as long as possible to maximise the benefit of allowing the skin to heal. Punch excision might be a complete treatment in itself or done before a resurfacing procedure.

Sometimes, a piece of skin from behind the ear is removed in the same way, to be used to 'fill' the original hole. This is a type of skin graft. The downside to this is that the skin colouring and texture from the graft may be different and therefore look less natural.

Surgical excision

This is where a dermatologist or surgeon cuts out a whole area of skin and sutures together a large section of atrophic scarring with a neat line that is easier to diguise.

Subcision

A fine needle is used to gently 'poke' around the area beneath the original scar. The idea behind this is to loosen any tightened collagen fibres, helping to release them and allow the scar to 'loosen' a little. The action of poking around may, itself, help to encourage more collagen regrowth in the area, helping it to re-plump. Like punch excision (see above), this can be done before undergoing other laser or chemical scar treatments.

Injectable dermal fillers

Collagen or synthetic types of collagen are injected directly into the area to help it plump out. An anaesthetic cream or gel is applied to help numb the area. Try to find a practitioner who has plenty of experience in doing this procedure. This will usually need topping up every few months, although it is reported that over time the frequency of injections needed may reduce.

Punch elevation

Deeper box-car scars can be treated by removing the original scar using the punch excisor (see above) but the removed area is lifted to the top of the skin and stuck in place using a special skin glue and steri-strips. The advantage of this is the ideal match in skin colouring and the need for only one procedure rather than a graft.

Treating rolling scars

Rolling scars respond best to subcision (see above) as it helps to loosen the tightened fibres at a deeper level. Other options might include a Dermaroller® (see page 133), chemical peels or laser resurfacing (see pages 130–1).

Other scar treatments

Dermabrasion

This method of treating scars was used for many years by surgeons. Now considered quite old fashioned, it has largely been replaced by laser resurfacing (see pages 130–1). However, if you are offered this type of treatment, it's useful to understand how it works. Dermabrasion is where the top layers of skin are removed by an instrument called a dermabrader. This will be carried out under general anaesthetic and involves literally sanding away the skin, which can be very bloody and messy. Recovery can take several weeks and the skin needs careful post-operative care to reduce the chances of infection.

Micro-dermabrasion

Available from beauty salons, this type of machine-operated device can be excellent at rejuvenating the skin and helping improve the appearance of mild scarring. It does not, however, penetrate the lower levels of skin, which is where deeper, longer-lasting scars are found. The operator will use a hand-held head attached to a machine. Micro-particles such as zinc or crystal are fired under controlled pressure onto the skin, in effect blasting it. This will lift the top layers of dead skin cells and then remove them by sucking them away. Sometimes a diamond-tipped head is used instead, which is claimed to deliver better results because of its ability to give a high 'polish' to the skin. Micro-dermabrasion is a bit like a super-powered vacuum cleaner that leaves the skin softer and more plumped in appearance. The downside is that it will need to be used regularly as the results are never permanent.

There is an increase in the choice and variety of home-based micro-dermabrasion kits. These vary in quality and price. Results will probably be noticeable but not long-lasting, and they are unlikely to give the same effect as salon-based options.

Laser treatments

There are two main types of laser treatment. The first, known as ablative lasers, will burn away top layers of skin to a precise and carefully measured depth. The other type, non-ablative lasers, will not damage the top layers of skin; instead, it tricks the skin into believing it has been injured, encouraging a self-healing response. If you are thinking about laser resurfacing, both types have their positive and negative sides. Each option needs to be given as a course of treatment and will usually be expensive (costs are rarely covered under the NHS).

Ablative lasers: These will literally remove the outer layers of the skin, burning away scar tissue and causing collagen to change. This results in a tightening effect, which then makes the scar less visible. Examples of ablative lasers include carbon dioxide and erbium:YAG but other types are available. Like dermabrasion (see page 129), this type of procedure will leave a bloody scar because the skin has been removed (albeit to very precise, carefully measured levels) and the resulting scab will need to be carefully looked after to prevent secondary infection. The layers are removed by using the laser beam to heat the skin, which in turn evaporates water in the skin cells.

Initial results of this treatment may seem far better than the final appearance. This is because the skin will swell in response to the laser. Some people are then disappointed when the skin has settled. This type of laser will affect the skin colouration cells (melanin) so the skin will always need to be protected in the future. The procedure may not be recommended for skin types 3–6 (see box on page 119).

Non-ablative lasers: These lasers are more suitable for treating milder scarring and sun damage. They trigger the skin to believe it has been injured, and to send out the body's immune cells to start healing. This healing process can help to re-stimulate collagen. Although this type of laser treatment can be uncomfortable (similar to having an elastic band flicked on the face) it will not require any 'down-time' – a period of recovery for post-operative wound care, such as after ablative lasers. An anaesthetic gel or cream can be used to help reduce any discomfort. There are a few different varieties of non-ablative lasers available. These include mid-infrared lasers and the two visible light lasers, the pulsed dye laser (PDL).

Chemical peels

These have been used for many years and are available in different strengths according to the depth of the scarring. Milder peeling agents can be used to give a general skin 'boost' but will do little to help scarring. Chemical peels allow the top layers to be removed, revealing fresher skin beneath. Some milder peels include alpha hydroxy acid (AHA), a chemical that occurs naturally in foods such as sugar, and lactic acid, which is found in milk.

Stronger peels that penetrate more layers of the skin are usually TCA (trichloroacetic acid) and come in concentrations ranging from 20–50 per cent, depending on how deep it is required to penetrate. TCA peels are more suitable for darker skins up to skin type 6 (see box on page 119). Usually the skin needs to be 'prepped' using a milder peeling agent such as an AHA. This will not give a one-off result and, like many other options, it will be necessary to use it regularly to maintain results.

A phenol peel is the strongest that can be safely used. This penetrates the skin to the lower levels, giving a better result. However, the downside is that it may need to be given under general anaesthetic, which carries its own risks. It will also create a scab on the skin that requires ongoing care and maintenance to ensure it doesn't become infected. This peel leaves the skin requiring future sun protection at all times.

Surgical facelift

This is clearly a drastic option and is not endorsed as a scar treatment in itself. It may help stretch the skin to help reduce the appearance of scars. Only a surgeon will be able to give advice on this option, which will require an expensive operation.

Micro-needling

This involves using a gadget, such as a Dermaroller®, to stimulate collagen, either in a salon or at home. It looks similar to a cotton reel covered in fine needles approximately 1mm long, attached to a handle to help it be rolled easily over the skin. Although simple, the design is quite sophisticated and usually made of stainless steel.

The device is rolled gently over the skin, and although it may tingle, it should not draw blood. The more often it is used, the better and longer-lasting the result, so it is recommended to be used daily. It is also reported to be helpful to allow the skin to absorb more from gels and creams by creating tiny openings in the skin surface, so it could be used in conjunction with other acne or scar treatments.

Disguising Acne Scars

While the ultimate aim of treating acne is to reduce the chances of getting scars, this is not always possible. Many scars will fade over time, leaving little or no permanent marks. However, as we have seen, some scars are deep and may require surgery or invasive procedures to help remove the damaged skin. Anybody either waiting for their scars to fade or undergoing treatment can use skin camouflage. This is still a relatively unknown choice, for several possible reasons:

- ○ It is perceived as being 'make-up' and therefore excludes all those who would not normally wear it – men and children.
- ○ It is not usually recommended, nor fully understood as an option, by healthcare professionals. This is usually because they don't know enough about it.

○ Access to an expert in skin camouflage is available in many dermatology departments through the British Red Cross (see page 255), although it varies around the UK.

See Chapter 11 for in-depth information on how skin camouflage works, whom it's for and how to use it.

Although scarring may be unavoidable for some people, for others it can be prevented by taking swift action to proactively treat acne as soon as it appears. Some might consider scarring to be a result of failed treatment, but despite our best efforts it may simply be impossible *not* to get some scars. Treatment options are mostly expensive and may be quite invasive, but technology developments may see more choice in the future.

CHAPTER SEVEN
ACNE AND POLYCYSTIC OVARY SYNDROME (PCOS)

Polycystic ovary syndrome (PCOS) is a condition where the ovaries contain a large number of cysts. Although the cysts are harmless, the condition can cause symptoms such as weight gain, irregular periods and acne. It is surprisingly common, especially among Asian women; reports suggest up to 52 per cent of women of south Asian origin in the UK may have signs of PCOS.[1] Other estimates suggest up to 20 per cent of women who are obese or overweight may have undiagnosed PCOS.[2]

There is a well-established link between PCOS and acne. However, women with acne are still not routinely investigated for PCOS, even though they may also have other symptoms associated with this condition. If any of the following symptoms are present, it is advisable to ask for a referral for a painless ovarian scan:

- ○ Acne – some doctors suggest that acne concentrated around the chin area may be more closely linked to ovarian disorders
- ○ Hirsutism (excessive hairiness) – this describes hair growth patterns more commonly seen in men, such as in

the moustache or beard areas. This can also be recognised in pubic hair that grows towards the navel
○ Hair loss on the scalp that may start with thinning on
the crown

Women with the above symptoms may have higher than normal
levels of male hormones (androgens). This is known medically as
hyperandrogenaemia. A blood test can measure levels of androgen in the blood to see if a woman is likely to have PCOS. Other
signs of the condition include:

○ Irregular periods, especially cycles that last more than
33 days
○ Failure to ovulate at all (known as anovulation)
○ Reduced fertility
○ Inability to lose weight – this is more likely to manifest
itself in the classic apple shape, in which larger amounts
of abdominal fat are stored

What are Polycystic Ovaries?

*The following information has been adapted from an article written
for the Acne Support Group by Dr Helen Mason, a scientist special-
ising in PCOS.*

In a normal ovary, a number of small fluid-filled sacs called
follicles begin to grow at the beginning of each menstrual
cycle. Each follicle contains an egg. As the cycle progresses,
one follicle will become the largest or dominant follicle, and will
go on to ovulate when it reaches about 2 cm. This happens at
mid-cycle which, in a 28-day cycle, is 14 days from the first day
of menstrual bleeding. As the dominant follicle grows, it causes

the other follicles that were around it to get smaller and gradually disappear.

In a polycystic ovary, twice as many follicles start to grow each month as in a normal ovary. We do not yet understand why. For various reasons in some women the dominant follicle does not grow and therefore the group of follicles does not get smaller and disappear. Gradually, the number of follicles increases to give the appearance of a polycystic ovary.

The link between having acne and your ovaries may seem odd at first, but the ovaries are a major site of production of one of the hormones that has a direct effect on the skin. These small, fluid-filled sacs consist of several different layers, each of which does a different job. The egg sits in the fluid in the middle and is surrounded by cells called granulosa cells. These cells produce the female hormone oestrogen. As the follicle grows it makes more and more oestrogen.

Surrounding the granulosa cells is another layer, which is called the theca layer. This layer makes the 'male' hormone androgen (testosterone). This then passes to the granulosa cells where it is converted into oestrogen by a chemical reaction. All of the oestrogen made in the ovary comes from androgen. However, not all of the androgen passes into the granulosa cells, and some gets out into the blood. In women with polycystic ovaries the theca layer makes a little more androgen; and in addition the granulosa cells are not working very efficiently converting it into oestrogen. This means that a little more androgen gets into the bloodstream. This then has effects on the skin in terms of hirsutism (hairiness) and increased oiliness and acne.

Testosterone levels are measured in women suspected of having this syndrome, but there is not always a direct link between the level of testosterone and the degree of acne or hirsutism. Other factors are involved, some of which are discussed further on.

Hormones that come from a gland below the brain called the pituitary control the growth and development of the follicle and the process of ovulation. There are two of these hormones: the first is follicle stimulating hormone (FSH) and the second is luteinising hormone (LH), which is involved in ovulation. Together they are called gonadotrophins. FSH stimulates the granulosa cells to make oestrogen. LH stimulates the theca cells to make androgen, as well as being involved in ovulation. The gonadotrophins may be out of balance in women with PCOS and so they are also usually measured.

The co-ordinated production of FSH and LH is dependent on signals sent from the ovary to the pituitary gland. One of these signals is oestrogen and the other is the hormone produced after ovulation called progesterone. Because the ovary is not working normally, both of these signals may be disordered in PCOS.

It seems likely that PCOS is passed down through families and so, although it doesn't become obvious until puberty, it is something that you were born with. Many patients have sisters with the same condition. What actually goes wrong in the ovary, we do not understand. Advances are being made continually and this may change in the next few years. Although PCOS can't be cured, it is possible to treat the symptoms in many women, which includes improving acne.

Treating PCOS

If you have regular cycles and your acne is not too severe, then you may be advised to take a standard contraceptive pill. The pill acts by reducing the pituitary production of gonadotrophins, which decreases the output of androgen by the theca. The oral contraceptive is composed of two hormones, oestrogen and progesterone.

One problem is that, in some preparations, the progesterone component may act like an androgen itself and make the problem worse.

One of the most effective treatments is cyproterone acetate (see Chapter 3, pages 72–4). This is an anti-androgen which reduces androgen output and is also able to block the effects of androgen on the skin. It is usually taken in the form of an oral contraceptive (Dianette®), as it is very important that a woman does not become pregnant while on this treatment. The beneficial effects of cyproterone acetate on acne are often quite rapid. The effects on hair growth will be slower because of the slow growth cycle of the hair.

Other options might include a course of treatment with a GnRH antagonist. This may be in the form of a 'sniffer' or given as an injection. This drug stops the pituitary gland making gonadotrophins, which then stops the output of hormones, including androgen, by the ovary. Although this may be an effective treatment for acne, it cannot be used for very long because of the side-effects. Because your ovaries will stop working, it is the equivalent of temporarily going into the menopause. You may experience symptoms associated with the menopause such as hot flushes and vaginal dryness. Prolonged use would cause the breakdown of the bones also found after the menopause.

Alternatively, Flutamide is a pure anti-androgen and may be given in cases where there has been no response to cyproterone. Spironolactone is a drug used extensively in the USA (mostly because they do not use cyproterone acetate) which may occasionally be prescribed for acne in the UK.

Losing Weight

One of the most important things to do if you have PCOS is to keep your weight down. There are several reasons for this. First, the amount of fat in the body will affect the level of testosterone acting on the skin. A proportion of testosterone is carried in the circulation attached to a protein called sex hormone binding globulin (SHBG). The testosterone attached to this protein is not able to exert its effects on the skin. The amount of SHBG in the blood decreases as your weight increases; less testosterone is therefore bound and more is free to act on the skin. Second, fat is a site of hormone production. The more fat you have, the worse the hormone imbalance will be.

One of the reasons women with PCOS gain weight easily is that they are better at preserving calories than women with normal ovaries. After a meal, a lot of calories are burnt off by the liver in the form of heat. This goes by a rather long name: 'postprandial thermogenesis'. This literally means 'after meal heat generation'. This is reduced in women with PCOS, meaning that fewer calories are burnt. Unfortunately, in effect, this means that you have to eat fewer calories than someone with normal ovaries to keep your weight down.

There is an even more important reason to watch your weight. It is becoming clear that some women with PCOS have a problem with their insulin and sugar balance. This means that they may be at an increased risk of developing diabetes in later life. The best way to avoid this is to have a healthy diet that is low in fat and sugar and to take regular exercise. During exercise the sugar is taken out of the blood by the muscles, keeping levels low.

Keeping to a low-glycaemic index (GI) diet may have a particular benefit for women with PCOS. This type of diet can help reduce insulin levels. Simple carbohydrate foods have a high GI. These foods, such as highly refined sugars, cakes and breads, are rapidly broken down during digestion and release glucose (sugar) quickly into the bloodstream. This stimulates insulin production, which in turn seems to upset the glands that regulate hormones. Foods that have a low GI break down slowly during digestion and release glucose into the bloodstream gradually, which does not cause the insulin surge and hormone response. Low-GI foods include proteins and complex, unrefined carbohydrates such as oatmeal.

Reducing insulin levels by diet is a relatively simple process. Insulin is stimulated mainly by carbohydrates in our diet, not proteins or fats. A low-GI diet where the amount of refined carbohydrates is restricted can be very beneficial in controlling PCOS and keeping the side-effects, including acne, at bay.

Foods to avoid include:

○ White bread, bagels and baguettes
○ White pasta
○ High sugar-containing cereals
○ White rice
○ Chips

Reducing the GI in a diet may take a little getting used to and may not give fast results but can be worth the effort. Try keeping your own diary to log changes and diet successes (or failures). Support this with a photo-log to record overall improvement of the skin.

CASE STUDY – SARAH

Being told I had PCOS came as a shock. I thought your acne had to be really bad and you practically needed a full beard before you would be taken seriously. I had the scan which revealed I had PCOS and was prescribed a course of treatment that involved taking a pill for certain days of the monthly cycle and then adding in more for the rest of the month. I was, however, told that I shouldn't expect the treatments to cure my PCOS but help with the symptoms.

By the third day of taking the tablets I experienced a migraine which was so bad I had to have the next three days off work. It was awful. I stopped taking the medication and decided to stick with conventional acne treatments. I would worry about any subsequent infertility at a later stage – I had plenty of time to make those decisions.

It took a while to get my skin under control but it did get better. I had other symptoms of PCOS like facial hair growth, which was really depressing, but I decided to bite the bullet and pay for laser treatment, which was expensive but worthwhile. I then read that trying a low-GI diet might help PCOS and decided I had nothing to lose. I am usually rubbish at sticking to things, but really wanted to give it a try. It seemed to help. I also used agnus castas drops in water once a day, which is meant to boost our hormones.

Getting a diagnosis of PCOS helped me to understand about WHY I had acne and facial hair problems, and I decided to get on with treating my acne anyway. I went on to have two healthy children and never seemed to have the issue some women do with infertility. I count myself lucky and realise that while the diagnosis wasn't good news, I could at least do something to help with the symptoms. It really helped me to speak to other women with this condition at the charity Verity (www.verity-pcos.org.uk).

PART TWO

ROSACEA

CHAPTER EIGHT
WHAT IS ROSACEA?

What do W.C. Fields, Bill Clinton and Prince Charles have in common? The answer is a ruddy complexion that has mistakenly been attributed to a problem with alcohol. This is only one of the challenges facing people with this condition. Many have never heard of it and assume their red face and flushing is merely a sign of aging, something they have to 'put up with'. While there are undoubtedly more people over the age of 40 who have this condition, there are still others who are in their early 20s or 30s who have it, yet because they don't know what it is, they may never receive a diagnosis.

A red face, and especially the nose, is the most common sign of rosacea (pronounced ROSE-AY-SHA), a skin condition described as far back as 1899 in a textbook on dermatology by Dr Norman Walker. Dr Walker wrote: 'the disease is often uncharitably attributed to alcohol, but all must be familiar with at least slight cases of the disease in tee total friends'. It is shocking that, over a hundred years later, this condition is still not widely understood.

So what is this mystery disease which affects up to 1 in 10 people in the UK?[1] The typical symptoms of rosacea include:

○ Facial redness, most commonly covering the nose and cheeks
○ Spots
○ Extreme sensitivity to temperature changes
○ Flushing and blushing

Leaving rosacea undiagnosed may lead to worsening of the symptoms in the future. More complicated and unwanted problems include enlargement of the nose (luckily rare) and severe broken veins or permanent redness. Some doctors estimate that up to 50 per cent of people with rosacea may also have symptoms in the eyes. For some it is possible to have rosacea only of the eyes with no other visible signs on the face. Complications associated with rosacea of the eyes often remain undiagnosed and untreated, risking serious (although extremely rare) consequences for the vision in later life.

Having a red face can be far more than just superficial. It can feel painful, sore, inflamed, swollen, tender, and as if the face has blown up in a volcanic eruption, boiling hot one minute, then settled the next. It can leave the skin feeling so sensitive that it cannot even tolerate water. It can be as if the face has taken on a life of its own and little can be done to halt its changes.

The good news is that this book will help you to discover that you *can* take control of your skin and, most importantly, how you feel about it. It may not be simple or straightforward, as some people with rosacea find that despite their best attempts it is difficult to fully control the symptoms. This section will help you to identify your own triggers, and show you how to log and keep control of them in the unique rosacea skin diary on pages 194–5. You will also understand that the choice of cosmetics needn't seem so perilous if you follow a few simple rules. The truth about skin camouflage (see Chapter 11) will be a revelation for men and women alike – once you realise how well it can hide facial redness, you'll be hooked.

Developments in the last 20 years have made a significant impact on rosacea patients' lives. We live in hope that funding for research into this common condition will continue, although the reality is that while far more 'serious' and 'life-threatening' conditions demand most of the money for medical research, rosacea still sits near the bottom of a very large pile. What science already understands about rosacea is that it can be managed well with a combination of treatments and lifestyle adjustments.

Rosacea can affect so many aspects of daily life, from interrupting sleep to influencing the choice of job, hobby or lifestyle. However, the basic rules about rosacea are:

○ If you let rosacea control your life, you will be a victim to it.
○ If you get the control back yourself, you will never be a victim to it.

If you haven't already received a diagnosis from your doctor or nurse, you should start by checking your symptoms in the quiz section (see Introduction, pages 5–6). Rosacea can be confused with other conditions, and for this reason the advice in this section can only be applied to diagnosed rosacea. Once you have identified your type of rosacea, you can follow the treatment guide on both self-help and prescribed treatments. Allow this book to be your companion during your search for the best treatments, skincare and advice you need to help keep rosacea symptoms at bay.

Understanding Rosacea

Many doctors use medical jargon to describe the different signs and symptoms of rosacea. For this reason, these terms have been included in this section. If, however, you are not sure what the doctor is telling you or feel unsure of the diagnosis or recommendations they make, always ask them to repeat and write down what they have told you.

What are the symptoms of rosacea?

Rosacea is usually one or more of the following symptoms:

○ Acne-like spots (papules and pustules, like red and yellow spots seen commonly in acne)
○ Red rash on the face (butterfly shape over the nose and cheeks)
○ Broken veins, especially on the nose and cheeks
○ Swollen, tender skin
○ Extremely sensitive or highly 'reactive' skin, with a tendency to flush easily
○ Dry, red or gritty feeling eyes
○ Enlarged, swollen nose

The classic sign is a band of redness that covers the cheeks and nose, but this may not always be present. However, any redness is usally symmetrically patterned (both horizontally and vertically), meaning that redness or a rash of small bumps or spots on the chin will usually be seen on the forehead, and a rash on one cheek will usually be found on the other. Only rare cases present symptoms in an unsymmetrical pattern.

Although doctors may prefer to categorise rosacea into mild, moderate or severe, it is quite possible that a person could have mild symptoms one day and more severe flare-ups the next. Alternatively, the severity of each symptom may vary. For example, someone might have moderately red cheeks and a mild case of swollen tender skin but their eyes may be severely affected.

How it feels to have rosacea

A lot of time is dedicated to describing what rosacea looks like, probably because it is usually a visually diagnosed condition.

However, some people have reported that while their visual symptoms appeared fairly mild, their experience of pain or discomfort was very high. However severe your rosacea, it is possible to feel any of the following sensations:

○ Burning
○ Stinging
○ Itching
○ Tenderness
○ Rawness
○ Soreness
○ Pain

If you feel any of these on a regular basis, be sure to tell your doctor or nurse. You may be advised to take painkillers to help control these symptoms. Other ways of reducing the severity of these symptoms are covered on page 180.

Other causes of flushing

Many women of menopausal age might experience hot flushes that affect not only the face, but the whole body too. These are triggered by the hypothalamus in the brain, which is also called the 'heat regulating centre'. This is similar to a thermostat which, triggered by menopausal changes, has been set slightly too low, tricking the brain into believing the body is too hot; the brain responds with a flush in an attempt to cool the body. The hormone oestrogen is responsible for stabilising the hypothalamus, and it is the reduction in this during menopause that triggers hot flushes. Hormone replacement therapy (HRT) may help control this type of flushing.

WHAT IS A BLUSH?

Frequent blushing is a typical sign of early rosacea but is it fair to assume that everyone who blushes will develop rosacea? And what is the difference between a flush and a blush? These are just some of the mysteries that surround blushing. A blush used to be considered charming in a lady, showing that she was demure and 'of good standards'. However, facial blushing in modern society can feel anything but charming or positive. For some it can be an endless cause of embarrassment and social disability.

A survey revealed that 45 per cent of people with rosacea found flushing to be the worst symptom of their condition, and 13 per cent reported they avoided any type of socialising because of this.[2]

The words 'blush' and 'flush' often get confused, but their meanings are basically the same: to turn red on the face, neck or ears. The upper chest can also be involved. This is accompanied by a feeling of intense heat in the same areas. Blushing is usually completely involuntary, meaning the muscles inside the blood vessels of the affected areas are prone to widen, allowing more blood to flow through them without any conscious effort. The redness usually disappears fairly quickly. Factors (other than rosacea) that can bring on blushing include:

O Illness, such as a high temperature or emphysema

O Emotions – these can range from love, embarrassment and self-consciousness to stress, rage and anger

O Heat – following exercise or walking into a hot room on a cold day

It has been suggested that blushing is a kind of 'unconscious apology' we make when we have done something that has caused us to feel embarrassed. However, for many people who experience frequent attacks with no apparent reason, this explanation may seem far from the truth.

In very rare cases a disorder known as 'carcinoid syndrome' can be the culprit for facial flushing. The symptoms of this serious condition include episodes of red flushing of the face lasting about 20 minutes, accompanied by sudden diarrhoea and stomach cramps. The usual cause of this syndrome is a tumour and will need urgent medical attention. If in any doubt, consult your GP.

Who is likely to develop rosacea?

The true cause of rosacea is still unknown, although numerous theories have been suggested (see below). However, we do know that some people are more likely than others to get rosacea for the following reasons:

○ One or both parents had diagnosed rosacea.
○ Their skin is type 1 or 2 on the Fitzpatrick scale (see page 119) – the classic Celtic skin types.
○ They are prone to blushing or flushing.

There is an exception to every rule, and it is not impossible to develop rosacea in skin colouring types 3 to 6. However, in these skin types the change in skin colouring is less obvious and other changes may also be harder to detect. Some doctors may fail to investigate because it might be assumed that rosacea doesn't happen in these individuals. Whatever your skin type and colouring you deserve to have your symptoms taken seriously, so rosacea should not be ruled out just on the basis of this.

Rosacea affects both men and women. It seems to be more common in women, although some men's apparent resistance to 'trouble' the doctor because of skin problems might be the real reason for the higher number of females diagnosed. It occurs mainly after the age of 30. However, some people develop it in their early teens or twenties, and others may not notice the first signs until well into their later decades.

FAST FACTS

○ Rosacea's appearance can change daily.

○ It is possible to have remission that can last months, or years.

○ Symptoms may include flushing and burning.

○ No one really knows why rosacea happens.

What Causes Rosacea?

In the quest to delve deeper into understanding the causes of rosacea, many theories have been proposed, with varying degrees of evidence behind them.

A vascular disorder?

Because tiny facial blood vessels are involved, it has been suggested that rosacea might be due to a problem with blood circulation. Flushing is a result of a sudden rush of blood to the face, and rosacea is associated with this symptom for the majority of people. The fact that so many people find their rosacea worse when they become stressed has also led some to believe that the vascular system working overtime is to blame. Some doctors have treated patients with 'off label' medication (not used for the indication for which it was licensed) that is also prescribed to patients who need to keep blood pressure reduced.

Skin mites?

It has also been suggested that a microscopic skin mite called *Demodex folliculorum* (which is found on most people's skin) might be responsible. These mites feed on dead skin cells. It is suggested that people with rosacea have many more of these mites than those who don't. It could be an interesting coincidence or something worthy of further research.

Lymphatic failure?

Facial swelling is due to an increase in blood flow during flushing, and this in turn leads to tissue fluid accumulating in these areas. This fluid cannot be drained quickly enough by the lymphatic system, causing the redness associated with rosacea. The skin tissue becomes thicker because of this trouble with drainage (this is called angiogenesis). This could explain why some people recommend manual lymphatic drainage (see page 179).

Helicobacter pylori?

This strange sounding but commonly found bacterium colonises the gut and is responsible for causing inflammation of the stomach lining and problems such as peptic ulcers. Small studies offer conflicting findings on whether this is also responsible for rosacea. It is interesting to consider whether antibiotics commonly used to treat *Helicobacter pylori* also happen to knock out the symptoms of rosacea, or if there is a stronger link suggesting that the bacterium is responsible for the rosacea. Some doctors believe that this is a red herring, however, and that this link should be discounted.

Diagnosing Rosacea

According to a panel of dermatology experts, rosacea has three degrees of severity.[3] While rosacea can be a progressive condition, meaning it starts off fairly mildly and progresses to a more severe disease, it is not always this easy to predict.

Primary features

To be diagnosed with rosacea, a person will have the presence of one or more of the following signs, located on the central face area. They may be transient (not long lasting) and any of them can occur in isolation. While these are common symptoms of rosacea, having one of them doesn't necessarily mean you have the condition:

○ Flushing (also called transient erythema) with a history of frequent blushing or flushing
○ Non-transient erythema – persistent redness of the facial skin, the most common sign of rosacea
○ Papules and pustules (papulopustular rosacea) – red papules with or without accompanying pustules (yellow, pus-filled spots), often appearing in clusters (blackheads are not a common sign of rosacea)
○ Telangiectasia – tiny broken veins and capillaries, especially on the cheeks and nose

Secondary features

○ Burning or stinging sensations, with or without scaling or dry skin

O Plaques – raised red patches

O Dry appearance – central facial skin may be rough and scaling, similar to dry skin associated with eczema. This may also occur with another condition often confused with rosacea, seborrhoeic dermatitis (see pages 160–1). These symptoms may be associated with burning or stinging sensations, and can be caused by irritation rather than the disease process

O Oedema – swelling due to a build-up of fluid – may accompany or follow prolonged facial redness or flushing. Sometimes soft oedema may last for days or be aggravated by inflammatory changes. Solid facial oedema (persisting hard, non-pitting oedema) can occur with rosacea, usually as a result of the papulopustular type. Swelling can occur without the appearance of any redness

O Ocular (eye) manifestations – these are common and range from symptoms of burning or itching to signs of conjunctival hyperemia (redness of the tissue that lines the inner eyelid) and lid inflammation. Styes, chalazia (cysts in the eyelid), and corneal damage may occur in many patients with rosacea. The severity of ocular manifestations may not be proportional to those of the skin

O Peripheral location – rosacea has been reported to occur in locations other than the face. Rosacea in peripheral locations may or may not be accompanied by facial manifestations

O Phymatous changes – when the skin thickens and gives a bulbous appearance. Rhinophyma (enlargement of the nose) is the most common form, but other phymas may occur

The primary and secondary rosacea features described above often occur together.

Rosacea subtypes

There are subtypes of rosacea that show more prominent symptoms.

Erythematotelangiectatic rosacea

This long word basically translates as red skin with blood vessels. It is mainly characterised by flushing and persistent central facial swelling. The appearance of telangiectases (broken thread-like veins) is common but not essential for a diagnosis of this subtype. A history of flushing alone is common among patients presenting with this type of rosacea.

Papulopustular rosacea

Papulopustular rosacea is characterised by persistent central facial redness with papules or pustules (red and yellow spots) or both in a central facial distribution. However, papules and pustules may also occur in other areas of the face so this often resembles common acne, except that comedones (blackheads) are absent. Burning and stinging is reported by patients with papulopustular rosacea.

Phymatous rosacea

Phymatous (thickened skin) rosacea often occurs on nasal tissue and can be seen in an enlarged nose (called rhinophyma) which is most often attributed to heavy drinking. However, skin thickening rosacea may occur in other locations, including the chin, forehead, cheeks and ears. It is twelve times more common in men than in women.

Ocular rosacea

The diagnosis of ocular rosacea should be considered when eyes have one or more of the following signs and symptoms:

○ Watery or bloodshot appearance
○ Foreign body sensation (feeling there is something in the eye)
○ Burning
○ Stinging
○ Dryness
○ Itching
○ Light sensitivity
○ Blurred vision
○ Reddening around the eye socket or of the eye itself
○ Blepharitis (inflammation of the eyelids)
○ Conjunctivitis (redness of the eye)
○ Stye (a lump on the eyelid)

Some patients may have decreased vision, caused by corneal complications, but luckily this is rare. Treatment of rosacea alone may be inadequate in terms of lessening the risk of vision loss resulting from ocular rosacea, and an ophthalmologic approach (referral to an eye specialist) may be needed.

Ocular rosacea is most frequently diagnosed when skin-based rosacea signs and symptoms are also present. However, skin signs and symptoms are not necessary in order to have a diagnosis of ocular rosacea. Limited studies suggest that ocular signs and symptoms may occur before usual skin symptoms in up to 20 per cent of people. Approximately half of patients experience skin lesions first, leaving 30 per cent experiencing both manifestations simultaneously.[4]

Neuropathic rosacea

This is a recently recognised type of rosacea that is yet to be officially adopted by dermatologists. However, this is a real problem for many people with rosacea who seem to slip through the net of other, more common variations of the condition. This type of rosacea causes bouts of long-lasting burning and pain that, for some people, seem to be semi-permanent. For these people, it's like the nerves around the areas usually affected by rosacea are firing off pain signals following exposure to the common rosacea triggers; this is why it is called neuropathic, meaning 'pain from nerve signals'. Why the skin reacts like this is still not understood, and treating it can be very challenging. Using suitable pain control and reducing or stopping exposure to triggers as quickly as possible are the first and obvious treatment routes to pursue.

CASE STUDY – GEORGE

My eyes had been bothering me for a couple of years – they had been watering, sore and itchy. I thought I had all-year-round hay fever and took antihistamines until I realised that they weren't working. It was uncomfortable more than anything else. My wife used to get eye drops for me from the chemist and they were okay but didn't do wonders, and the problem would always return. My doctor was stumped and it was only after I insisted that I be referred to an ophthalmologist that I discovered I had a condition known as blepharitis, which was actually more like rosacea of the eyelids – very strange. He put me on a course of antibiotics and prescribed a cream, and within weeks it had almost completely gone. I wouldn't say I was cured because I do get trouble from time to time, but when it seems to be playing up I make sure I get my cream from the doctor. I was amazed that I was told I had rosacea of the eyes – my wife has had rosacea for years and I know what that looks like but my symptoms were only really in my eyes.

Rare types of rosacea

Just as with acne, there are less common types of rosacea that will require a dermatologist (skin specialist) to diagnose and treat. The two key types are rosacea fulminans and rosacea conglobata.

Rosacea fulminans

This is also called 'pyoderma faciale' and looks like a cross between severe acne and severe rosacea. It will usually start very aggressively, appearing in a severe form almost overnight. Unlike other forms of rosacea, it doesn't appear in men. It will usually be fairly short-lived compared to the length of time people commonly experience rosacea. This condition is confined to the face and will not be associated with flushing or greasy skin. Treating pyoderma faciale requires help from a dermatologist who may use a combination of treatments. These are likely to include the strong acne treatment isotretinoin (see pages 74–82).

Rosacea conglobata

This is very similar to fulminans but may bear a closer resemblance to severe acne (without the comedones). The deep sinus tracts may need to be injected with corticosteroids to help reduce their size. It may be necessary to have some of these surgically removed if using steroids fails to work. First-line treatment for this aggressive type of rosacea will be isotretinoin in most cases (see pages 74–82).

When is it not Rosacea?

Because rosacea has a range of symptoms it can be confused with similar looking skin diseases so it's vital to receive a correct diagnosis from a GP or nurse to be sure. The description of rosacea outlined in the section above is quite extensive and there are usually clear areas of difference between rosacea and the conditions described below.

Perioral dermatitis

Perioral means 'around the mouth' and dermatitis means 'inflammation of the skin', which helps to explain how and where it appears. A typical pattern of this condition is seen in the tiny 'halo' or gap left between the lips and the bumps and red lumps. Like typical rosacea there may be variations in severity, ranging from a mild rash to severe itchy lumps that occur around the mouth, nose or even the eyes. This condition is thought to be triggered by using steroid creams or ointments, which may also ironically be used to treat it. The inappropriate use of steroids may prolong this condition as well as have no long-term beneficial effect, with symptoms usually returning as soon as steroids are stopped. However, other factors can trigger this condition, including make-up and skincare products. Hormonal influences, such as being premenstrual or taking the contraceptive pill, might make it worse. Treatment options usually include a course of antibiotics.

Systemic lupus erythematosus

Also called 'lupus', this is an auto-immune disease that can affect almost any system in the body. It is as if the body has become allergic to itself, resulting in a breakdown in the ability to function properly. This can produce pain, inflammation or, in the worse cases, organ damage. As it can be widespread it is not always easy to identify to begin with, although physical symptoms such as a butterfly rash on the face will usually present with other signs such as general fatigue or flu-like symptoms. Lupus requires long-term management and treatments that vary greatly from those for rosacea.

Contact dermatitis

This is an allergic reaction seen in the skin. The allergy can be to almost anything. Some people may never discover what has caused the reaction, which usually results in itching, swelling and redness. However, common culprits may be cleansers, make-up, shaving products, hairsprays or perfumes. It might be helpful to cut out products used on the area to see if there is any improvement. The area affected may be small or large and will not usually follow the symmetrical pattern of rosacea.

Seborrhoeic dermatitis

This is often mistaken for rosacea because of how it looks, appearing red and patchy. It is an inflammatory disease caused by overgrowth of a yeast on the skin called *pityrosporum*. It causes the skin to become scaly and flake off. This is associated with dandruff. While we might expect dandruff on the scalp, it can spread to other areas of the face. It is possible to have both rosacea and seborrhoeic dermatitis at the same time. This condition often responds well to an anti-yeast shampoo such as Nizoral®. If it has spread to the facial area, then allow shampoos to run over the face as this will help to keep it under control. However, to get the best from these types of shampoo, they need to be left in contact with the skin for approximately five minutes. Take care to avoid contact with the eyes. Like rosacea, this condition can get worse with stress.

Photosensitive dermatitis

Some people's skin can become extremely sensitive to ultra violet (UV) light. This can happen as a result of burning in the sun or using products on the face. Others may not be able to find the source of their problems. The typical sign of photosensitive dermatitis is skin redness and extreme sensitivity, which is why it might be confused with rosacea. Photosensitivity tests can be carried out to confirm the diagnosis. (See Chapter 12 for further tips.)

Acne

Part 1 of this book covers acne in more detail. Spots commonly seen in rosacea will also be common in acne. Some doctors still insist on referring to 'acne rosacea', which only adds to the confusion. However, key differences between the two can be summed up in the table overleaf.

Acne	Rosacea
Comedones (open and closed blackheads)	No comedones
Greasy, oily skin	No greasiness, usually prone to dry skin
Can affect any area covered in sebaceous glands	Mostly confined to the central face region, rarely affecting the body
Not usually progressively worse	May get progressively worse if left untreated
No symmetry to outbreaks	Usually symmetrical

Rosacea Triggers

Unlike acne, rosacea seems to be sensitive to triggers that can make it worse. This may be a vital key to controlling rosacea. Understanding what may trigger an 'attack' or worsening of rosacea as soon as possible may help avoid many of its negative effects, including depression and feeling out of control.

Triggers for rosacea include diet, lifestyle and medication, and may be a combination of all or some of these factors. There are also other triggers such as the strong influence of weather/temperature and changing seasons. Some of these are obviously beyond our control, but there is still a lot that can be done to help reduce exposure to any trigger factors identified.

The importance of finding out what makes your rosacea worse cannot be emphasised enough and should be one of the priorities in a treatment plan. Few doctors will discuss or consider a treatment plan for rosacea, but this is a multi-pronged approach that looks at every aspect of life that may affect rosacea, not just treatment alone.

There are undoubtedly many potential triggers for rosacea and the following list will be far from complete. However, the best advice is to use it as a guide, applying the principle that being aware of the impact of the various aspects of daily life will allow you to keep an open mind to a selection of possibilities. It is likely that there will not be one single trigger, but many small triggers that combine to make the problem.

A survey carried out in 2005 identified the following most common triggers:

Emotional stress

Nearly 75 per cent reported that stress alone was responsible for their flare-ups. Many added that their rosacea made them feel more stressed, which created a vicious circle. Episodes of stress have been known to trigger rosacea instantly, and the flare-ups can last until the stress is under control. Understanding this connection could be helpful to identify the time to start treating the skin in advance of a flare-up.

CASE STUDY – LAUREN

I had never had a problem with my skin; in fact, I used to be complimented on how clear it always looked. In my mid-40s I was often mistaken for someone in their 30s. Everything changed though when I went to Africa to undertake some research for a book I was writing. I was then in my late 40s and looking forward to an exciting adventure. However, while out on a visit, I became involved in what can only be described as an ambush. The small group of tourists I was travelling with was held captive for three days. This was exceptionally distressing and my stress levels skyrocketed so badly that I instantly developed the most severe facial redness and spots I have ever seen. It happened as soon as we were taken and didn't settle until I was safely back home in the UK and well into a long course of antibiotics. My doctor thought it was some sort of emotional reaction to the stress I had experienced and suspected it was rosacea. I had never heard of it but upon researching more about it I discovered it is possible that stress can play a part. In my case it was more than just a part – it was the only cause of it. I keep my skin under control with a mixture of gels and tablets and stick carefully to a caffeine- and alcohol-free diet, which I find helps greatly to reduce the flares-ups.

Hot or cold weather

Nearly 70 per cent cited extremes of temperature as their trigger. Cold weather leaves the skin feeling extremely tingly for some. A sudden change in temperature, coming from outside cold into a centrally heated building, is particularly challenging. Hot weather will encourage a flushing response, and in those predisposed to flushing this can obviously make rosacea far worse. Prolonged exposure to sun could also damage the skin and make rosacea worse.

Wind

In the survey, 52 per cent of respondents reported that windy weather made rosacea worse. Some added that having to avoid the wind meant dropping outdoor pursuits or having to give up a job that involved working outdoors.

Spicy foods

Under half (42 per cent) of respondents reported that spicy foods triggered their rosacea. This figure seems rather low as this is commonly believed to be the culprit in rosacea. Spicy foods can trigger a flush response that contributes to rosacea symptoms.

Alcohol

Drinking alcohol made rosacea worse for 63 per cent of respondents. Some additional comments in the survey reflected society's belief that rosacea happens to alcoholics, and this leaves people with rosacea often feeling too embarrassed to drink openly in public. Many people with rosacea will avoid alcohol altogether for this reason.

Hot baths

In the survey, 39 per cent felt hot baths (or saunas) made their rosacea worse. Any excess steam should be avoided wherever possible as this triggers a flush response.

Skincare products

Make-up or skincare products were blamed by 56 per cent for their flare-ups, although many were unable to say which particular brand or type was the culprit. Some people added that they tried to avoid any products that contained alcohol or might be astringent.

Hot drinks

The heat from a hot drink (or soup) in a cup held close the skin can worsen rosacea. This has the same effect as being in a steam bath or sauna. In the survey, 28 per cent reported this as a trigger factor. It is worth noting that caffeine has been shown to make no difference – it is the heat that is important.

Certain foods

Although 44 per cent blamed particular foods, the range of food and food groups was hugely varied, including:

○ Tomatoes
○ Cheese (except cottage cheese)
○ Spinach
○ Yoghurt
○ Plums
○ Raisins
○ Vinegar
○ Yeast-containing foods
○ Chocolate
○ Marinated foods

Medicines

Some medicines may act as vascular dilators, meaning they change the flow of blood around the body. These may make the symptoms of rosacea worse. They might include alpha- or beta-blockers for treating high blood pressure or heart problems, or medicines that contain steroids, especially those used on the skin.

Unknown triggers

Interestingly, nearly a quarter (23 per cent) couldn't pinpoint what triggered their rosacea. It could also mean that some people don't believe they have any triggers.

Multiple triggers

It is possible that someone could have one, two or many of the common triggers described above, which could make it hard to manage everyday life. It is not known how many people have multiple triggers, but anecdotally it is likely to be around half of all people with rosacea. Some people are careful to avoid anything that makes their skin worse, following strict diets or making lifestyle adjustments.

Appreciating the variety of causes and triggers for rosacea can put you back in the driving seat. It gives you the power to seek suitable treatments and avoid anything you believe makes it worse. While there is no 'cure-all' when it comes to rosacea, there are many avenues to explore. Try to stay positive and remember that however bad your flare-ups may be, there will be options to help keep the skin under control and irritation and discomfort to a minimum.

CHAPTER NINE

TREATING ROSACEA

The good news is that rosacea can be effectively treated for most people. However, like treating acne, it will require patience and perseverance as there are no quick fixes or guaranteed cures. This section deals with many different aspects of treating the varying signs and symptoms but is, most importantly, a guide to help you feel back in control of your skin. If you cannot cure your rosacea, it is vital to find a way to keep it under control. Also, because rosacea may be made worse by a variety of triggers discussed in the previous chapter, these need to be considered and addressed at the same time as taking or using treatments.

Managing Your Rosacea Treatment

Part of the frustration of rosacea is being unable to predict its course. Some doctors have even suggested that it may 'burn itself out', which doesn't seem to ring true for many people who have endured symptoms for years. It is fair to say that this condition may be difficult to 'cure' (this word is unfortunately rarely used when talking about many skin problems) but with work it can be controlled. It might be helpful to consider rosacea as a 'spectrum' condition; this means it has many degrees of severity matched by an equal number of symptoms, all of which can happen in different combinations.

TOP HOME REMEDIES FROM PEOPLE WITH ROSACEA

○ Pop open a vitamin E capsule and apply the contents to drier areas.

○ Apply a soothing mask of pure aloe vera, available from various health food shops or directly from aloe vera suppliers.

○ Use a mild exfoliator, such as glycolic acid, which may target the demodex mite (a tiny organism that apparently digests dead skin cells within the hair follicle and is reputed to be responsible for rosacea in some people).

○ Ultrasun sunscreen has a wide range of sunscreens and has been reported to be very helpful for those who work outside all day, in all weathers.

○ Mix aloe vera gel with a few drops of lavender and tea tree essential oils twice a day, apply sparingly to the face and allow the skin to absorb this natural soothing gel.

○ KCN makes a range of skincare products for people with rosacea (www.calminskincare.co.uk). This company knows all about the particular problems of rosacea as the owners have had it for years themselves!

Treating rosacea may end up being a step-by-step process full of successes and setbacks. As this is not unusual, it might be helpful to anticipate it to avoid the common disappointments that being set up for a 'cure' can give. To prevent the frustration of trying a range of treatments and then forgetting what you have tried, it might be useful to keep a personal rosacea treatment plan: a log of treatments used and their results. This treatment plan might also include:

○ Self-medication (from the pharmacist or supermarket)
○ Any alternative or complementary medicines

○ Dietary changes or supplements
○ Skincare products

Keep a log of what, how much and how long anything was used, and what results it gave (good or bad). Taking this one step further, it might also be productive to include other aspects of daily life that may affect the skin, such as:

○ Lifestyle – outdoor pursuits, hobbies or sports that may make you sweat (or freeze!)
○ Stress levels
○ General wellbeing – are you sleeping well, eating healthily?

Information gathered on all these aspects can help to build an in-depth picture of your life and the factors that may be helping or hindering your recovery from rosacea. You may wish to use the rosacea treatment plan diary template on pages 194–5.

Treating Different Rosacea Symptoms

Treatment for rosacea will usually depend upon the symptoms you experience. Some commonly prescribed antibiotics, for example, may have a positive effect on inflammation but will do nothing (or little) to help with flushing. Once your rosacea has been diagnosed, seek treatment that is best for that type (see previous chapter for a description of each type). If you have a subtype of rosacea, such as ocular rosacea, see the treatment advice starting on pages 180–1. Otherwise, decide which one or more symptoms from the list below you have for guidance on appropriate treatment options:

○ Flushing/blushing
○ Broken or spider veins
○ Inflamed, red or spotty skin

Flushing/blushing

The key to controlling this symptom of rosacea will be to reduce the frequency and severity of attacks. It will help if you are able to identify any underlying triggers (as listed on pages 162–7) that you feel are linked to your blushing.

Laser therapy

Lasers can be very useful for treating rosacea symptoms associated with redness, such as flushing and red veins. There are two main options: pulsed dye laser (PDL), which uses a flash of light that targets colouring on the skin, and intense pulse light (IPL), which uses a non-laser light.

Psychological help

There may be some straightforward psychological reasons for blushing, such as shyness, but blushing itself links back to feelings of embarrassment and self-consciousness, which makes a person feel shyer. It can therefore be a vicious circle. There are ways to help break this cycle, which are built around tackling these feelings head-on:

○ Cognitive behavioural therapy (CBT) – a 'talking treatment' designed to help reveal how your problems began and how you may unconsciously help keep them going. It works on three aspects of behaviour – what you think, what you feel and what you do – breaking them down to help you identify any links. Once you have found these links, they can be changed through conscious choice.

○ Breathing techniques – a variety of breathing techniques may be helpful to maintain a sense of control and provide a distraction from anxiety.

○ Neuro-linguistic programming (NLP) – a recognised selection of techniques to help address underlying feelings and unhelpful behaviours associated with blushing. This can include hypnosis or visualisation techniques.

○ Yoga – many varieties work on deep breathing and relaxation exercises and can be easily continued at home. Be aware that some types of yoga can be fast-paced and therefore far from suitable for help with people prone to blushing.

All of these techniques will take time to master and require effort and focus. The rewards can be substantial for many people and, although the blushing may not completely disappear, the severity can be reduced and often controlled. Practitioners in the above therapies, plus a range of other types of psychological/relaxation-based specialists, can be found in local directories or online. Check they are registered with a professional body or organisation before committing to any treatments.

Endoscopic thoracic sympathectomy (ETS)

This is a drastic, risky and major surgical option that is usually reserved for those who are experiencing severe periods of prolonged blushing. ETS was first pioneered to help hyperhidrosis (excessive sweating). The operation involves entering the body through the side of the chest cavity, locating the sympathetic nerves and cutting selected nerves responsible for blushing. If the blushing occurs on both sides of the face, both sides will need to be operated on, meaning two incisions. The major risk of this operation is that it carries the chance of affecting other nerve functions in the same area and can result in losing nerve functions, such as the ability to sweat, to have goose bumps or for the pupils to dilate, among others.

Undergoing ETS surgery requires very careful consideration of all the risks and benefits. Talk to your GP for initial advice. This procedure may not be available on the NHS in all areas of the UK.

CASE STUDY – STUART

I couldn't function any more with the amount of blushing I was experiencing. I was socially crippled and hadn't left the house in three months when I decided I just had to do something once and for all – my rosacea was completely ruining my life.

I read somewhere about this operation you could have where surgeons sever the nerves that feed the blushing response, located under the armpit. I must confess I didn't relish the idea of the operation, and the hospital made it absolutely clear that there were very strong risks. I agonised over the decision for months and really tried to get myself out and about a bit more to see if I could face the world. However, the first time I did venture out (which was only to my local pub with a couple of mates) an acquaintance shouted over to me, 'Don't worry about lighting the fire tonight, we've got Stuart here to keep us warm.' Although I tried to laugh it off it really hurt to have my problem turned into a joke. This comment was the final straw and the next day I arranged to go back to the hospital to discuss the surgery. Because it wasn't considered important enough, I had to pay for the operation myself and it was really expensive, so my decision to go ahead reflected just how desperate I was.

On the day of the operation I was really nervous but excited at the idea of clearing my problem up so I went into the op feeling hopeful. The surgery went ahead as planned and although I felt groggy after the op, I couldn't wait to see if it had made a difference. The surgeon said he felt it had gone well but we wouldn't know for sure until I had recovered from the operation. A week later I noticed that one side of my face was perfectly clear. Unfortunately, the other side was just as it had been before and I can't tell you how odd that looked to see a half-red, half-normal-coloured face in the mirror. I was even more embarrassed but encouraged because at least it had worked on one side. I returned to my surgeon who said that this can happen and there was no guarantee they could get the other side working properly, but they were going to have to re-operate.

Luckily the operation was a complete success and the redness/blushing I used to have has now completely gone – it was like they had soldered some wiring and literally cut the connection to my face.

Broken or spider veins (telangiectasia)

Broken or spider veins are a common sign of rosacea. They usually occur because the skin has been exposed to prolonged flushing attacks that have caused the tiny capillaries beneath the skin to break, leaving a purplish or red thread-like mark behind (this is also why they are referred to as 'thread veins'). They can appear around the nose, chin and cheeks as well as other areas of the body such as the ankle or knee. Treating these can be quite straightforward and usually successful.

Pulsed dye laser

This effective treatment works by firing a yellow beam of light at the affected blood vessel through a fibre optic cable. At the end of this cable is a hand-held, pen-like device, which sends a rapid pulse of light directly onto the affected area. This penetrates less than 1 mm into the skin and the light is then absorbed by anything that is coloured red. Broken veins are predominantly this colour so they quickly heat up. This heat is responsible for destroying the blood vessel, leaving a bruise in its place. This bruise will usually heal within 10–14 days. To help counteract the heat, a cooling gel or jet of air is used. This makes it a more comfortable experience, although some people have reported it is a little like having an elastic band flicked at the face.

The skin will usually need to be well protected from sunlight during the course of treatment and for several weeks after it is finished. Darker skin types (skin types 3 or higher on the Fitz-patrick scale, see page 119) may find it leaves darker or lighter patches of skin.

Creams

You can buy creams that promise varying degrees of success with spider veins. However, be aware that some of them are nothing more glamorous than haemorrhoid creams (not usually recommended for the face), which are used to shrink blood vessels. They will probably need to be used for at least a few weeks before you notice any effect.

Cautery

In this procedure an electric current is passed through an instrument that resembles a flattened needle to heat it up. The heated end is then applied to the broken veins and causes a small burn, which then encourages healing. This healing process should resolve the broken veins, but is not always successful and might leave a small scar. Get advice on this option from someone experienced in using it regularly.

Skin camouflage

This is not a treatment but is excellent for any skin colouring and can be used during or after other treatment options. It will successfully conceal broken veins as they are flat. (For more information on skin camouflage see Chapter 11.)

Inflamed, red and spotty rosacea

This can be fairly straightforward to treat. The first point of call is your GP or nurse, who can prescribe a variety of treatments. These include the following:

Antibiotic tablets

These are also referred to as 'systemic antibiotics', meaning something that is taken by mouth. The particular type of antibiotic that is prescribed for you will depend upon several factors:

○ Previous use of antibiotics – any known allergies or bad side-effects from previous courses are noted in your records, and these types will therefore be avoided. Some people are resistant to specific antibiotics, meaning the antibiotic will have no effect.
○ Severity of the condition – the dose and type of antibiotic can be adjusted, starting with a higher dose or lower dose. Your doctor or nurse will decide which is best.

Antibiotics that can be prescribed include:

○ Tetracycline
○ Doxycycline
○ Erythromycin
○ Lymecycline
○ Minocycline

Taking any type of antibiotic can give excellent results, but may need to be used long term for continual benefit. Interestingly, the reason they work is because they reduce inflammation. Once they are stopped the symptoms usually return. This is why, as with treatment regimes for acne, it might be wise to discuss a gradual withdrawal of antibiotics rather than suddenly stopping, which might cause a flare-up. This 'stepping-down' can also be combined with starting a course of topical antibiotics, in effect switching over.

Antibiotics taken by mouth, if taken over a long time, may cause stomach upsets or thrush. Tell your doctor or nurse if this worries you or if you are prone to these complications.

Topical antibiotics

Treating rosacea with topical gels, creams or lotions can give results as good as using antibiotic tablets. It also avoids the possible complications of stomach problems and thrush.

The range of topical antibiotics available includes:

○ Metronidazole
○ Erythromycin
○ Clindamycin
○ Tetracycline
○ Low-dose doxycycline Efracea®

Azelaic acid

Doctors can now prescribe non-antibiotic treatments for rosacea that appear to give similar results. There is the added benefit of avoiding/reducing antibiotic resistance problems. Azelaic acid is derived from barley, wheat and rye. Clinical trials have proven it to be as good as antibiotics. It is available in 15 or 20 per cent strengths (Finacea Gel® or Skinoren®, respectively), but it cannot yet be obtained without a prescription in the UK.

Treating Subtypes of Rosacea

Phymatous rosacea (swollen skin)

This is where the skin becomes thicker, especially around the nose, leaving it appearing large and bulbous (rhinophyma) (see

Chapter 8, page 155). The thickened skin can be treated with several options:

Isotretinoin

The usual starting point for treating swollen skin is the strong acne medication isotretinoin. This has been shown to give some improvement, but just how and why it works for rosacea symptoms such as phymatous is not fully understood. The list below gives the most common side-effects but is not comprehensive. You are more likely than not to experience one or more of these side-effects. Therefore, it is important to anticipate them and take steps to ensure they are counteracted or carefully managed:

○ Dryness of the nose, eyes and lips. Sometimes the skin may become cracked and very dry, which may lead to bleeding in these areas.
○ Muscle aches and pains
○ Sensitivity to sunlight
○ Risk of depression
○ Serious risks of abnormalities, including death to an unborn baby

In acne, isotretinoin is likely to cause a flare-up of the condition, but in rosacea it is harder to predict what side-effects to expect. Keep moisturisers and emollients handy to use as and when the skin becomes excessively dry, and allow up to six weeks before you expect to see an improvement. Just as in patients with acne, it is likely you will need to be monitored by the person who prescribed it; this includes an obligatory pregnancy test if you are a female of child-bearing age.

More information on this drug can be found in Chapter 3 (pages 74–82.)

Laser ablation or electrosurgical excision

The ablative types of laser (those that 'cut away' the skin) can be useful to help shave away the thickened skin and restore it to a normal appearance. The most commonly used of these are the erbium:YAG and/or carbon dioxide lasers, which can 'shave' away micro levels of the skin without causing too much bleeding (if any) or going too deep so that healing is compromised. A very effective alternative is electrosurgical treatment, where an electric wire is used to cut and reshape the nose under a local anaesthetic. They can give long-lasting results and probably offer one of the best options for more severe cases of rhinophyma. To find out if lasers are a suitable option, begin by speaking to your GP about the options for an NIIS referral.

Dermabrasion

This technique was used more frequently before the advance of lasers, which are now the treatment of choice. Dermabrasion is a messy operation, involving removing top layers of skin using a sanding technique. This isn't as accurate as a laser and produces a lot of blood from the area being treated. Bleeding can increase the risk of infection and healing time compared with the more gentle lasers. For this reason it is not routinely offered in the UK.

Manual lymphatic drainage (MLD)

MLD is a type of light skin massage without the use of oils. It claims to help reduce the symptoms of facial swelling by removing excess fluid. It is non-invasive, relaxing and painless. Once shown the technique, you can do it yourself at home.

Neuropathic rosacea (painful nerve-associated rosacea)

This can be one of the hardest types of rosacea to treat because it is not associated with as many physical signs as some other types.

It may be barely visible but extremely painful. Managing the pain may require the combined efforts of a neurologist (a nerve specialist), a dermatologist and your GP. The main key with this type of rosacea is to identify any triggers and to work to control or reduce them as quickly and as much as possible. For people experiencing this, it may be impossible for them to bear any type of lotion or cream on the skin including, in some extremes, water. Ways to help relieve this include:

○ Use a tepid water spray to help cool the skin.
○ Try cotton wool pads soaked in distilled water and gently squeezed. You can store these in a bag and keep them cool in the fridge. They may help to soothe any burning pain.
○ Carry a hand-held fan to help keep cool.

Some people have found vasoconstrictors helpful. These drugs contract blood vessels that are responsible for giving the burning sensation. Some migraine medication available from the pharmacist might help. Ask the pharmacist for further advice.

Ocular rosacea (rosacea in the eyes)

Ocular rosacea requires early treatment to prevent the condition deteriorating (see Chapter 8, page 156, for a description of symptoms). Start by bathing the lids with a mild solution of sodium bicarbonate, which can help calm sore inflamed eyelids. You could also use damp cotton wool pads placed over the eyes to soothe any burning and to help keep swelling down. Store these in the fridge in a plastic bag and throw them away after use. Camomile tea bags soaked in cold water, squeezed and then stored as the cotton wool pads add extra soothing benefits for some. If these home remedies don't help, then other further treatments usually involve steroid eye drops to reduce the inflammation and some of the irritation in the eye. Artificial tears also help by lubricating the eye (ask for a brand without preservatives). These are usually available directly from your pharmacist.

If these fail to keep the symptoms under control, visit your GP or nurse for advice. They can prescribe a course of tetracycline antibiotics. These work by reducing the inflammation in the eye and around the eyelids. Studies have shown that the early use of tetracyclines can prevent the onset of further complications.

Don't put up with eye pain or discomfort or accept that you 'just have to live with it'. If necessary, you may have to be referred to an ophthalmic specialist by your GP or nurse for further investigations and treatments. In emergencies, visit the eye casualty department; this is usually within the eye department of your local hospital. Eye problems that are left untreated may worsen over time.

Complementary Rosacea Treatments

Just like those treatments that claim to help acne, alternative and complementary therapies for rosacea often lack scientific evidence, making doctors wary of their potential benefits. However, many people have given positive feedback on a wide range of remedies.

Acupuncture

This has been used to help overcome rosacea, but evidence is still not forthcoming on its proven benefits. It is unlikely to make rosacea worse, although some people have reported that their skin flushed during treatment and returned to normal shortly afterwards. (For more information, see Chapter 4, pages 96–7.)

Aloe vera

This is a popular choice for many people with a variety of skin complaints. Aloe vera is a type of succulent plant that is easy to grow at home, making it an ideal home-grown remedy. Simply snap off a stem and apply the liquid from the centre of the stem directly to the skin. Be sure to use the transparent fluid and to avoid the yellow/green sap that also oozes from a snapped stem as this is likely to irritate the skin. Alternatively, aloe vera can be bought from health food shops or supermarkets in a variety of options including powders, drinks and capsules.

Burdock root

Burdock root aids natural detoxification and there are claims that it has helped people with rosacea-like symptoms for centuries. A teaspoon of the dried root can be added to 250 ml water, put in a saucepan and brought to the boil, then allowed to simmer until it has reduced by half. Aim to have one cup a day.

Calendula

This marigold extract can be taken in a tincture or capsule formula. It is an ancient treatment for inflammatory conditions.

Camomile tea

There are claims that camomile tea can help the circulation and may therefore reduce the severity of flushing. It can also help restore a sense of calm and relaxation. This is widely available from most stores and health food shops. A cloth soaked in cooled camomile tea can help to soothe the skin and can be used as a compress.

Chrysanthellum indicum cream

This cream contains a herbal extract that appears to strengthen capillaries, so helping to reduce facial redness. One study showed encouraging results when this was compared to a placebo, conclud-ing that it is effective and well tolerated in moderate rosacea.[1]

Digestive enzyme supplements

If you also suffer from indigestion problems, pancreatic enzyme supplements taken with a meal may not only help the digestive problems but can improve rosacea symptoms too.

Evening primrose oil

This is a popular remedy, particularly for women with rosacea, and is well known for its natural healing powers for a variety of condi-tions. Packed full of natural fatty acids that help the body fight inflammation, it is widely available and harmless to take.

Flaxseed oil

Another of nature's oils, high in 'good' fats that help the body to heal and repair itself.

Ginger

This is claimed to help reduce redness and inflammation. It is available as teas and powders and can be added to hot drinks. It helps to reduce cholesterol and may have blood-thinning properties. Be aware that ginger can interact with warfarin (blood-thinning medicine).

Liquorice

This can be used on the skin or taken internally. Consult a herbal-ist for advice on using this herb. Some people have reported eating liquorice to help their rosacea, but no hard evidence of its benefit can be found.

Milk thistle

Milk thistle helps to detoxify the blood. It protects and enhances liver function, which is believed by some to contribute to the cause of rosacea. The liquid form is recommended as it lasts longer in the digestive system than the capsules. Milk thistle tea is unlikely to contain enough active ingredient to have the same effect as the liquid formulation.

Nicotinamide

This is a form of vitamin B3 available as a cream or gel, as well as in tablet form. The tablets are taken as supplements. The gel formula is currently marketed as 'Freederm® Gel' and is aimed at the young end of the acne market, although its gentle action means it can be tried on rosacea skin. It is excellent at calming redness and reducing inflammation.

Rosehips

Rosehips reportedly have a high vitamin C content. When fruit was scarce during the Second World War, mothers used crushed rosehips to keep up their children's vitamin C intake. High doses of vitamin C are claimed to help the body fight infection and inflammation. This common plant extract can be found in many formulations including teas, marmalades, drinks, powders and oils.

Tea tree oil

In acne problems, tea tree oil has proven benefits, significantly reducing inflammation. However, this oil can be highly irritating, especially to tender, sensitive rosacea skin types. Use it diluted by adding a few drops to daily moisturisers and water used to wash the face. If your skin is extremely sensitive, try a small patch test first.

Zinc

Zinc helps the skin to heal and recover from injury or disease. Most people should be able to get sufficient amounts in a balanced diet, but taking supplements might be helpful as long as you don't exceed 25 mg a day.

Managing Trigger Factors

The key to minimising flushing attacks is to identify what makes them worse. Once you know what these 'triggers' are, it's possible to take positive steps to reduce unnecessary exposure to them. It may not be easy to simply stop or completely avoid some of them, but a common-sense approach to keeping exposure to a minimum can help. Here is some advice on how to reduce some of the triggers.

Stress

This term may cover a lot of emotions. It isn't always caused by life-changing events as some people respond to stress more effectively than others. Some degree of stress isn't necessarily a bad thing; a bit of stress may help us to push ourselves harder, giving rewarding results. However, many people with rosacea find that stress can be a major reason for their skin getting worse, which, in turn, causes further stress. Following these three steps might help manage stress and break the stress cycle:

1) Try to understand what is causing your stress

Are you worried or anxious about something you have little or no control over? Or is there something you can do to positively change what is making you feel stressed? The key with stress, just

like managing rosacea, is to understand that you have the ability
to change how you feel. For example, you may feel stressed due
to moving house or changing jobs. You can't (or won't want to)
undo these changes, but you can change how you feel and react
to them. Managing stress may not always be easy, but it can be
possible to reduce it by knowing exactly what is making you feel
it. Break down what is stressing you into small bite-size pieces
and deal with each piece one by one. If there is nothing you can
do to change something outside of your control, then why let it
stress you?

2) Look after yourself

Being kind to yourself and taking time to think about relaxing and
unwinding will greatly help reduce stress. You can switch your
focus onto you and your feelings through visualisation techniques,
yoga, meditation or a relaxing massage. Ask yourself, 'Do I care
about myself enough?' The answer may reveal whether you need
to pay more attention to this area and take positive action towards
changing it for the better.

3) Take up a hobby

Hobbies and interests are all about taking a bit of 'me time' to
focus on a pleasurable activity. People with rosacea have reported
that taking up a new hobby has greatly helped reduce their stress
levels and given them a positive focus in life.[2]

Hot or cold weather

Experiencing extremes of temperature can easily trigger a dilation
of the capillaries as blood rushes around the face. These flare-ups
can also feel hot, even burning, and can be embarrassing to experience. Try to reduce sudden changes in temperature:

○ If you know when you arrive home in winter that the house will be hot, why not turn a radiator off in the first room you are likely to step into? This can reduce the sudden change from cold to extreme warmth. Give your skin a few minutes to warm gradually before entering other, more heated rooms.

○ If leaving a warm room to go into chilly weather, protect the face by wearing a scarf up around the cheeks, covering as much of the face as possible.

○ In hot climates, carry a hand-held fan to keep the skin cool.

Wind

Cold, biting winds can leave rosacea skin feeling raw, sore and burning. The obvious answer is to keep out of windy environments. If it is not possible to avoid wind, then the following may help:

○ For the best protection wear a scarf and a hat.

○ Some creams claim to help protect skin from the elements, but how well they will work against sudden changes of extreme weather has not been proven.

○ Some people recommend using Vaseline® (petroleum jelly) on their skin, as it acts as a barrier.

Spicy foods

Many types of spicy, chilli-containing food act as natural vascular dilators, meaning they increase blood flow, particularly around the face. In people with rosacea this will make the problem worse and can easily be avoided:

○ If you like spicy foods, reduce the amount of spices you add and eat this type of food less often.

○ If you are going to eat spicy food, take a cooling face spray or some cooled cotton wool pads soaked in water with you to use for any subsequent flare-up, and drink plenty of water with your meal.

○ Accept that if you like spicy foods and your skin doesn't, there will be times when one loses out to the other!

Alcohol

Alcohol also acts as a vascular dilator, bringing on a red flush that can make rosacea look worse. This is often why people with rosacea are unfairly mistaken for alcoholics. Wine, especially fortified wine, has more of an effect on rosacea than beers or spirits. If you enjoy a drink but want to keep any rosacea flushes to a minimum then be selective about what you drink, how much and how often. Here are some general tips:

○ If you are going to have alcohol, then either dilute your drink or take small sips.

○ Keep a good supply of any topical gels or creams that help with flare-ups, and be ready to use them after drinking alcohol.

Hot baths

Steam produced by any source seems to aggravate rosacea flushes so it makes sense to avoid steamy atmospheres as much as possible. Therefore, keep away from hot baths, steam rooms and saunas.

○ If you know you are not going to be able to avoid steam then have a cooled face cloth handy to keep over your face and continue to keep it cool with tepid water.

○ Turn down the temperature of your bath water and leave a window open for ventilation.

○ Switch to showers and lower the showerhead nozzle to keep hot water off the face.

Skincare products

A number of skincare products make rosacea far worse. In some people, skin products have actually caused their rosacea. Caring for rosacea skin is very challenging and requires a close look at ingredients and routines (for more on this, see Chapter 10). However, here are a few golden rules to help if you find that skincare products trigger or worsen your rosacea:

○ Look for products that claim to be suitable for 'intolerant', 'sensitive' or 'reactive' skin.

○ Avoid astringent toners.

○ If your skin feels hot and regularly has burning flare-ups, keep any moisturisers, face creams or sun protection in the fridge and use when cool to help soothe the skin.

Hot drinks

Hot drinks of any type will produce steam, which is the enemy of rosacea. Leave drinks to cool sufficiently so that the steam has reduced, and don't hold them around the face unless drinking from them.

EMERGENCY ROSACEA SOLUTIONS

There are two major issues with rosacea: heat, which is a result of flushing, and redness, which is a key sign of rosacea. Dealing with a rosacea 'attack' can be challenging as it may be prolonged and difficult to control. However, by working with the two key elements of heat and redness, it may be possible to regain some control.

HEAT

If getting hot makes your rosacea worse try carrying with you:

○ A pack of dampened cotton pads wrapped in plastic – use to cool the skin.

○ A facial 'spritzer' available from chemists or beauty salons – or make your own version by using cooled, boiled water in a small spray bottle.

○ A small hand-held fan – use to keep the face cool.

REDNESS

If it is not possible to avoid what makes your skin redden, try these tips:

○ Make sure you have supplies of prescription rosacea treatments with you to use to calm redness.

○ Apply a cold compress to the skin (as cold as your skin can tolerate).

○ If your skin turns red because of a link with embarrassment or other psychological reasons, invest time in learning some self-help measures to use in a potentially difficult situation. These might include visualisation or 'tapping' (part of emotional freedom technique or EFT) among others.

Medicines

Various medicines (either prescribed or over-the-counter) can make rosacea flushing worse. Medicines likely to cause problems include:

- ○ Viagra® – increases blood flow
- ○ Steroids used on the skin

Any decision to withdraw a medicine or stop suddenly should be taken in full consultation with whomever prescribed it.

MORE TIPS FOR DEALING WITH ROSACEA

None of these tips is proven to work for everybody and are just suggestions passed on by people with rosacea. A healthy, balanced diet is recommended so you should avoid cutting out food groups altogether.

- ○ Allow hot foods and drinks to cool slightly before eating or drinking. This can help people whose condition is triggered by heat or steam.
- ○ Try replacing cows' milk with soya or goats' milk. This can also apply to other dairy products such as cheese.
- ○ Avoid foods high in salicylic acid. This is an ingredient used in many over-the-counter acne medications. Fruits and vegetables are natural sources of salicylic acid, with fruits having large amounts of salicylates, particularly berries. Some herbs and spices also contain quite high amounts. Meat, poultry, fish, eggs and dairy products contain little or no salicylates. The highest content can be found in green peppers, olives, mushrooms, tomatoes, radishes, apricots,

blackberries, blueberries, dates, guavas, raisins, almonds and peanuts.

○ Colax colon cleansing tablets have received mixed feedback, with some people hailing them as 'a miracle'. Others, especially those prone to irritable bowel syndrome, may find the tablets aggravate their stomach.

○ Betaine hydrochloride and pepsin can help to calm the stomach, which in some cases may have a connection with rosacea flare-ups. These are available from health food shops.

○ Try to be as gentle as possible with the skin and don't scrub it too much. If you can get away with it, leave the skin alone as much as you can, and have a regular 'leave-my-skin-alone' day where you use nothing on it at all.

○ Avoid sun beds and sunbathing. Wear a wide-brimmed hat when out in any type of sunshine. The skin can burn even on a dull British summer day.

○ Avoid steroid creams. These may worsen rosacea and, in some cases, be responsible for the condition. If it is necessary to use a steroid cream, then use the lowest strength for the shortest period. Steroids can work quite fast to reduce inflammation but will not usually have long-lasting effects.

○ The widely used ingredient phenol, found in shaving creams and other products, may cause stinging and rashes.

○ The demodex mite, thought to be a possible cause of rosacea, has been treated with a medication used for scabies. This treatment is 'off-label', meaning it is not usually recommended. It must be used with great caution – once a week to begin with and only following a small patch test. Permethrin is the most recommended treatment and can be purchased from pharmacists without a prescription.

○ Some people have reported that anti-dandruff shampoo which is allowed to run down the face during a shower has helped improve their rosacea. This may actually point towards the condition being seborrhoeic dermatitis rather than rosacea (see pages 160–1). Avoid getting the shampoo into the eyes and leave it on the skin for as long as possible before rinsing.

Rosacea Treatment Plan Diary

People with rosacea may find their skin is better on some days than on others. The reasons for this may never be fully understood. To help identify different aspects of daily life that may have an impact on the condition of the skin it is a good idea to keep a diary. This will also help you to gain a sense of control and understanding of the condition. If your skin worsens for no apparent reason, the diary can help to track subtle changes that may have occurred in the days leading to the flare-up. Something as simple as a change in the weather or feeling stressed about world events can sometimes make the skin worse.

The key to managing rosacea effectively is to feel firmly in control. Use the template below as a sample to start your own daily log, which can help to build up an individual treatment plan. This diary can also be used to share information with your doctor and help banish any suggestion that 'you are making this up', which some doctors may be inclined to imply. This may be especially so if you experience a particularly 'good skin day' on the very day you visit your doctor or specialist. If it helps, include photographs as well. These will act as an excellent means of reviewing your skin.

You may photocopy this or adapt it for your own use.

	Food & Drink	Medication	Skin Products	Weather	Mood	General Activities
Sunday .... Skin (circle a number): **1 2 3 4 5 6 7 8 9 10** (1 = good, 10 = very bad)						
Monday .... Skin (circle a number): **1 2 3 4 5 6 7 8 9 10** (1 = good, 10 = very bad)						
Tuesday .... Skin (circle a number): **1 2 3 4 5 6 7 8 9 10** (1 = good, 10 = very bad)						
Wednesday .... Skin (circle a number): **1 2 3 4 5 6 7 8 9 10** (1 = good, 10 = very bad)						

	Food & Drink	Medication	Skin Products	Weather	Mood	General Activities
Thursday .... Skin (circle a number): **1 2 3 4 5 6 7 8 9 10** (1 = good, 10 = very bad)						
Friday .... Skin (circle a number): **1 2 3 4 5 6 7 8 9 10** (1 = good, 10 = very bad)						
Saturday .... Skin (circle a number): **1 2 3 4 5 6 7 8 9 10** (1 = good, 10 = very bad)						

CASE STUDY – CLARE

I used this diary for a whole year to help track my skin. At first I couldn't really get a lot from it – I just felt it was a bit of a chore. However, after a few months, when I looked back over the previous period I realised there were some interesting links that I hadn't spotted before and it felt empowering to understand this possible link. I discovered that whenever I spent time gardening my skin would flare up the following day and stay that way until I stopped my gardening sessions (because of rain and so on), yet the weather was not always sunny or warm, which I assumed would be the usual trigger. Although I suspect my flare-ups are linked to exposure to sunlight I have learned that it doesn't even have to be a bright day to affect me.

My way around this? I loved my gardening and found it therapeutic so I wasn't going to give it up because of my skin – instead I invested in a really good sunblock made by Calmin and bought a lovely wide-brimmed hat which I secured with a chin strap so it could withstand my head bobbing up and down. This really helped and my diary log reflected an improvement. I also discovered that eating tomatoes made my skin worse, something I had never noticed before. Cutting out tomatoes and using my new gardening attire seemed to do the trick, and all because of sticking to my rosacea diary!

PART THREE

CARING FOR ACNE AND ROSACEA SKIN

CHAPTER TEN

SKINCARE ROUTINES FOR ACNE AND ROSACEA

Caring for the skin should go hand in hand with using prescription treatments. For both men and women, it is sometimes difficult to find the right skincare to use alongside treatments for acne and rosacea. The more you know about your skin type, the easier it is to develop a successful skincare routine and to feel in control of your skin.

The skin functions at its best when it is moist, supple and well lubricated. It produces its own natural protective layer called the acid mantle. As the name suggests, this is slightly acidic, with a pH of 5.5. It is made up of a combination of moisture from our sweat glands and oil from our sebum ducts. If it gets disrupted, the skin becomes drier, more sensitive, sore and chapped. Dry weather, harsh winds, extremes of temperature and over-exposure to the sun can all make it worse.

The underpinning principle when using any type of skincare is to maintain, strengthen and avoid stripping the acid mantle. Many manufacturers market their products with this in mind, describing them as pH balanced. When products are described as being too harsh, it is because they strip off these natural protective layers.

Using everyday soaps designed to clean dirty feet and smelly armpits should be avoided on areas affected by acne and, particularly, rosacea. It is important to rinse soap off the skin but this can be difficult if the water is high in calcium. The best advice about basic everyday cleaning is to avoid harsh soaps and exchange them for gentle soap-free cleansers that can do a much better and kinder job.

Remember, the skin will eventually restore its own natural acidity. However, like most things, it happens more slowly the older you grow!

A Guide to Skincare Ingredients

Before going into detail about the wide range of skincare products, it is helpful to understand some basics about ingredients. You may not realise:

- O Under EU law, ingredients must be listed on packaging.
- O Unlike medicines, cosmetic ingredients do not have to undergo strict testing for effectiveness.
- O The percentage of active ingredients does not have to be included. Therefore, some acne or rosacea products may be marketed on a particular ingredient that is too small to make a difference.
- O Ingredients are listed in order of the highest content. So, if the active ingredient for acne or rosacea is number 11 out of 12, it is not likely to have a huge benefit.

Potential allergens

A recent amendment to EU cosmetic regulations included a list of 26 chemicals that must be declared within the ingredients if they are present in the formulation above the following levels:

○ 0.01 per cent in rinse-off applications such as shower
gels or shampoos

○ 0.001 per cent in leave-on applications such as creams
and lotions

The 26 chemicals identified as potential allergens, according to
their International Nomenclature of Cosmetics Ingredients (INCI)
name, are:

1. Amyl cinnamal
2. Benzyl alcohol
3. Cinnamyl alcohol
4. Citral
5. Eugenol
6. Hydroxycitronellol
7. Isoeugenol
8. Amylcinnamyl alcohol
9. Benzyl salicylate
10. Cinnamal
11. Coumarin
12. Geraniol
13. Hydroxyisohexyl 3-cyclohexene carboxaldehyde
14. Anise alcohol
15. Benzyl cinnamate
16. Farnesol
17. Butylphenyl methylpropional
18. Linalool
19. Benzyl benzoate
20. Citronellol
21. Hexyl cinnamal
22. Limonene
23. Alpha isomethyl ionones

24. Methyl 2-octynoate
25. *Evernia prunastri* (oakmoss) extract
26. *Evernia furfuracea* (treemoss) extract

It may (or may not) be helpful to watch out for these, remembering that they may be present in tiny amounts in some products. One person may react to an ingredient that has no effect on someone else. Rosacea skins are more likely to be 'reactive' so this list cannot be considered complete. Other potentially irritating ingredients that are slipped into a range of skincare and cosmetic products include:

Sodium lauryl sulphate

This detergent is commonly used in shampoos and cleaning products. It can cause irritation and is often used to deliberately irritate skin to test the benefits of skin protectors.

Mineral oil

This is a by-product of petroleum. It coats the skin, clogging the pores and leaving a plastic-like film behind. It can interfere with skin's ability to excrete, which is why it can make acne worse and cause sweat glands to become blocked. Baby oil is 100 per cent mineral oil!

Parabens

Parabens, such as methyl, propyl, ethyl and butyl paraben, are used as preservatives. They work by reducing microbial growth and therefore extend the shelf life of products. Although many products containing parabens do no harm, they should be avoided in rosacea skin types wherever possible.

Ethanolamines

Monoethanolamine (MEA), diethanolamine (DEA) and trieth-anolamine (TEA) are added to products to help stabilise pH levels. When exposed to oxygen/air they form nitrosoamines, which can be irritating and/or toxic.

HOW OLD IS A PRODUCT?

If you want to know how long cosmetics or skincare products can be used for, check the packaging. Under EU rules, the package must show how long (in months) a product is considered 'safe' to use before it needs to be discarded. Look for a pot-shaped design that has a lid removed (it looks like a container for false teeth!). Next to it will be the number of months, for example 30M, which means 30 months. Pots that allow a person to dip their fingers in are more likely to harbour germs than tubes or bottles that pour the contents out.

Basic Skincare Steps

It's hard to say if our caveman ancestors considered washing an important part of survival, but we do know that grease and grit can be an enemy to both acne and rosacea skin types. Part of caring for the skin should include three important basic steps:

○ Cleanse
○ Moisturise
○ Protect – against the sun

Although our skin may not need more than a gentle cleanse each day, acne and rosacea skin types deserve extra care. Even oily skin commonly found in acne types could benefit from an oil-free moisturiser, especially as many topical treatments for acne can leave the skin dry and sensitive. Protecting against the sun should be a common-sense approach for both skin types; in acne the sun may interact with some prescription medications, and in rosacea it may trigger a flare-up or make existing tender skin more sensitive.

Cleansing

This just means 'to clean' and should be the first step in everyday skincare for everyone, including men. However, when your skin is highly reactive, sore, itchy, greasy or spotty, this requires careful choice, although it doesn't mean you have to spend more money. What you want a cleanser to do is:

○ Remove surface dead skin cells to reduce pore blockages
○ Remove make-up or other facial products
○ Allow the skin to 'breathe'

Choice of cleansers

Advances in cosmetic science have seen the introduction of a variety of cleansers and implements (tools) to help achieve deep cleansing, but which are best? Currently the choice is as follows:

Facial cleansers: Available in gel/liquid or solid formulations such as cleansing bars. These are usually mixed with water and rubbed on the skin. These cleansers are also available as either a 'mix with water and wash off' variety or as a combined cream cleanser that you apply and then remove using a cotton cloth or cotton wool pad without rinsing. Some people prefer this one-step process, which can be used anywhere, not just at a sink! Fragranced soaps are designed for use on the body and should be avoided on facial areas, whatever the skin type.

Implements: These include facial brushes and woven mesh pads which are used together with facial cleansers. They work by exfoliating (removing) the top layers of dead skin cells and can leave the skin feeling smooth and 'buffed'. Be careful when using these on more sensitive skin types, although if used gently they needn't be too harsh or damaging. Keep their use to a minimum – twice a week should be sufficient.

Disposable facial wipes: Since baby wipes were first introduced their use has grown and spread across into the skincare and household markets. The fabric used is impregnated with various cleansing agents and can be used to remove make-up or as part of a cleansing routine. They can contain some astringent ingredients such as ammonium lauryl sulphate and ammonium laureth sulphate or alcohol, which can be harsh to the skin. The looser the weave on the cloth, the softer and less abrasive it will be to the skin. You'll be able to tell this by the amount of holes in the cloth; the more, the better. This type of cloth offers a 'wash on the go' option and can be useful for teenagers who might be averse to using water! Avoid the fragranced ones, which may irritate your skin.

Skin scrubs/exfoliators: These work by adding an extra component that provides an exfoliating surface, giving gentle friction to remove dead skin cells. Some of these are harsher than others. Although some are suitable for daily use (and marketed as such), it is not necessary to use one this often. Scrubs can be used twice a week for the same effect and will make the product last longer. Ingredients range from micro-bead technology (which just means tiny beads) to natural, everyday products such as oatmeal, apricot stones or walnut shells. Micro-beads are likely to be made of polyethylene, which are smooth and ball shaped and therefore kinder to the skin; crushed stones or shells may be too harsh as they have rough edges.

Some other types of exfoliators don't need to be rubbed into the skin as they will naturally remove dead skin cells in a dissolving action. These are known as either alpha-hydroxy acids (AHA) or beta-hydroxy acids (BHA) and have been used for centuries to help hold back the signs of aging. BHA is available in only one form, salicylic acid, and is widely used in acne products and some prescription medicines. It is fat soluble, meaning it will penetrate deeper to dissolve the oil in blocked pores. AHA is water soluble and more widely used in a range of skin products. It needs to be left on the skin to give the best results, so products containing AHAs don't usually work if they have to be rinsed off. Some products contain such small amounts of BHAs or AHAs that they have little benefit, so look for them being second or third on the listed ingredients.

Cleansing acne skin types

Removing greasiness and blocked pores is the key challenge for a cleanser. Washing with water alone is unlikely to achieve much more than a refreshing blast that will simply slide off the skin taking none of the oil with it. Therefore, acne skin needs something that will 'grip' the oil and penetrate the pores sufficiently to help loosen any blockages without removing the top layers of skin with it. Simple steps for cleaning acne skin types include:

○ Use a face cloth or clean hands to wash the face. If using a face cloth make sure it is washed at least once a week and leave it to dry thoroughly after each use.

○ Wash with a mild soap-free cleanser or face wash (watch out for cleansers that may be too mild as they fail to remove surface oil). Choose a cleanser designed for acne/greasy skin types.

○ Wash all areas usually affected by acne. Remember to include the neck, chest, shoulders and back (this is probably best done in a shower).

○ Rinse well to remove any remains of the cleanser.

○ Pat (don't rub) the skin dry.

Cleansing rosacea skin types

Cleansing this type of skin needs to be accompanied by the mantra 'gentle, gentle, gentle'. There are some people who are unable to tolerate even something as gentle as water on their skin, but luckily this is rare. One popular face wash range for people with rosacea skin is Cetaphil® as it is reported to be exceptionally gentle, even to irritated and sensitive skin. Anecdotal reports suggest that the routine of washing delicate skin as little as once a week solves the problem of irritation and doesn't over-dry it. A typical wash routine for rosacea skin types might be:

○ Use tepid water and a gentle face wash. Rub the face wash between both hands before applying to the usual areas, wiping gently.

○ Use a cotton wool pad soaked in tepid water to gently remove the cleanser.

○ Leave the skin to dry naturally, patting off any excess drips if necessary.

○ Spray with a cooling rosewater spritzer (be aware that these may be fragranced).

○ Apply any prescription facial gels at this point.

○ Leave for up to 10 minutes before applying moisturiser.

Moisturising

The aim of using a moisturiser is to reduce water loss from the skin. There are two main types: oil-in-water or water-in-oil. The oil-in-water moisturisers often contain humectants that work by attracting water from the lower levels of skin to the top, helping to keep it moist. At temperatures over 70 degrees Fahrenheit, they will also attract water from the atmosphere. Most importantly, they work as a barrier between the skin and harsh external elements. A commonly used humectant is glycerine.

Water-in-oil moisturisers work by forming an occlusive film, trapping water beneath. The balance between the ratio of oil to water will depend upon the skin type for which the product has been formulated. In general, 'normal' skin types will need an oil-in-water moisturiser, and drier skin types will need water-in-oil to boost moisture retention.

Acne skin types should avoid oil-containing moisturisers, but there is no reason why moisturisers shouldn't still be used. They can be very helpful to counteract the dryness of harsh acne products. Moisturisers for acne are usually labelled as oil-free, or 'non-comedogenic'.

Some useful moisturising tips for both rosacea and acne skin include:

○ Apply moisturiser after washing and after any medication, but before using any skin camouflage or make-up.
○ Leave the moisturiser to be absorbed naturally rather than rubbing.
○ Expect the skin to shine after it has been applied.
○ Rub it into your hands before applying to the skin, using a gentle patting motion.

○ To get more from your moisturiser, add a drop of lavender or tea tree oil, although be aware that tea tree oil
may be an irritant to more sensitive skin types – patch
test first if you are not sure.

Sun protection

Everyone should use sun protection, whatever their skin colouring or type. Even a cloudy day in the UK leaves skin vulnerable to
UV rays. Not only can these make rosacea worse, they also cause
changes in the skin that lead to signs of sun damage, such as
premature wrinkles and an increased risk of skin cancer. Although
UV radiation may help some people with acne, it should never be
considered a 'treatment' and still leaves the skin at risk of damage.

If you wear make-up, check to see if your foundation, powder
or tinted moisturiser already has an SPF (sun protection factor).
You will need to use a minimum of 15. It is easy to boost the SPF
by adding your own sun cream, especially if you are sensitive to the
sun. Either add a few drops to your foundation or tinted moisturiser before you apply it, or if using powders, apply on the face
and leave to absorb first.

If you are taking antibiotics, which can leave your skin more
sensitive to sunlight, use at least an SPF of 30 for darker skin types,
and up to a total sunblock for lighter shades. (See Chapter 12 for
more information on sun protection.)

Extra Treatments

Face masks

Face masks are usually of a paste consistency and are left on the
skin to work for up to 10 minutes. They may dry out during this

time, which is normal, and are then rinsed off to remove completely. These might best be considered a more indulgent aspect of a skincare routine, a treat rather than a part of your daily ritual. It's possible to make your own mask, which can be just as good as commercial ones, minus harmful chemicals and additives. They can not only leave the skin feeling refreshed, but also help to soothe burning, hot rosacea skin or calm red acne skin types.

Face masks for greasy skin types

○ Whisk an egg white until thick, then add one teaspoon of honey. Add one teaspoon of lemon juice and apply to the face, avoiding the eyes. Leave this on for 10 minutes before rinsing with warm water.

○ Mix one medium-sized, grated apple with five table-spoons of warmed honey and leave on for 10 minutes.

○ Mash half an avocado and apply to the face. Leave for up to 15 minutes before rinsing off. It will leave your skin feeling very soft.

Face masks for rosacea skin types

○ Purée half a cucumber, add a tablespoon of natural yoghurt and mix well. Leave on for up to 15 minutes.

○ For a really nourishing face mask mix one egg with one teaspoon of almond oil and one tablespoon of semi-skimmed milk.

Toning

A toner is used after cleansing and before moisturising. It may also be called a skin tonic, drench or spritz. Its aim is to refresh the skin. Toners, contrary to popular belief, don't close the pores. They work by irritating the skin sufficiently to swell the surface so the pores appear smaller. This is often a short-lived response. Although they may be astringent, they can be helpful for giving a 'deep clean' feel. They can also be used on their own as a cleanser, as they are particularly good at removing grease. Toners don't have to contain alcohol. They can be based on milder ingredients, such as rosewater or citric acid, which are more likely to be skin-friendly. If you wish to use a toner, then try a spray rather than something that is wiped over the skin.

Toners are quite controversial as many experts claim they are unnecessary and marketed as part of a three-step skincare process to improve sales. The choice to use them should be down to the individual.

Visiting a Beauty Counter

It's easy to think you are going to feel intimidated by a glamorous assistant who looks like she has never had a spot in her life, but this image may be unjustified. People who work on skin and beauty counters have usually been trained to give advice on their range of products, and many are passionate about their work. Where people's expectations may fall down is when they want advice on medical skin problems, such as acne and rosacea. These counter assistants are not usually qualified to give this advice.

The assistant will usually be keen to show you their range of products, but you should never feel intimidated or manoeuvred into buying anything you are not sure about. They will want to make the experience as pleasant as possible for you, and may invite you to try some of their products. While this is an excellent way of experiencing creams, lotions and make-up, people with sensitive skin may feel uncomfortable having their usual make-up removed and sitting in a public place. It may also lead to a flare-up of

TOP TIPS FOR VISITING THE BEAUTY COUNTER

○ Explain your skin problems and skin type, as well as any creams or lotions that you usually use on your face. This should affect their final recommendations.

○ You should give a new product time to settle on the skin to see if it causes a reaction or flare-up. Ask if the assistant can let you have samples to try at home. You could take a small clean pot with you.

○ Take your usual make-up remover or skin cleanser so you can do this yourself at the counter. This will save a potential bad reaction spoiling your experience.

○ Ask the assistant to show you how to use any products you buy. If necessary, get them to watch you do it yourself in a mirror so they can give you advice.

○ Take someone you trust with you to give you an honest opinion and reduce any feeling of being under pressure to buy.

○ If you are not sure about something you have tried, then go home with the product on to give you time to decide if it is suitable and non-irritating. Any beauty counter assistant who values their work will understand that this is likely to ensure you are a happy customer willing to return to buy the product if it is right for you.

○ If you are not happy with a product, especially if you feel it has not done what it claims to do, then send it back with a covering letter of explanation. Many reputable skincare companies will be keen to keep your business and try to help with other products in their range.

○ Trial and error is the best method – do ask for samples and allow for some successes and failures. Despite the best advice, we can all make the wrong decisions about skincare on occasions.

rosacea, so ensure that anything used on the skin is patch tested first, rather than applied all over.

Although beauty counters may look and feel like a strictly female domain, men will always be welcomed, especially as most of the counters in department stores sell a wide range of products that go far beyond purely cosmetic make-up. (For more information, see 'Skincare for Men', on page 213.)

CASE STUDY – EMILY

I have always been interested in skincare products because I have obsessed about my skin for as long as I can remember. I don't have a problem visiting a skincare counter to ask about make-up but I find it really difficult to talk about my acne problem with strangers. However, I was desperate for something, anything to try because my skin was particularly bad, so I gathered all my courage to ask a beauty counter assistant for advice. I was astounded when she told me that I looked like I had an allergy. She said she had a friend with a similar problem that ended up being an allergy to their pet rabbit!

I was very downhearted and left without buying anything because I just knew she didn't have a clue what she was talking about. I did, however, decide to try again at another store where I knew the staff were better trained about skincare. I was relieved to find a really sweet, helpful woman who told me she understood my problem because she had suffered from acne for years herself. She was full of good advice – the best of which was telling me to go to my doctor! She didn't even try to sell me anything. However, she did suggest that once my skin was getting better I should go back to her for some samples to try. I ended up spending over £100 just because she was so helpful. The products were great for what they were – which was skincare – and they worked really well with the antibiotic gel the doctor prescribed for me.

> I think the people on the counter are only as good as their train-ing and their enthusiasm for skincare. Don't be put off trying, but if you suspect someone hasn't a clue what they are talking about don't part with your money, no matter how sweet they may be!

Skincare for Men

Most of the advice in this chapter applies equally to men. The prob-lem for men is that few products on the market are aimed at them, and some of those that are contain highly perfumed ingredients.

Research suggests that men's skin is thicker and prone to being oilier than women's. This means that men need products aimed specifically at their skin type. However, there is still much to gain from using products for acne or rosacea skin types, regardless of whether they are specially designed for men or not. Look for the key ingredients that help to reduce acne, described above; if you have rosacea, seek fragrance-free and 'gentle on the skin' ranges.

Shaving

The obvious difference between men and women's skin is the need to shave the face. For people with acne this can be a very traumatic experience. Some men have reported they would prefer to grow a beard both to avoid the problem of shaving and to disguise spots. However, this needn't be necessary if you know how to shave properly.

Shaving tips for acne skin types

Ingrowing hairs occur when the hair is cut and regrowth causes the hair to curl back on itself or the hair fails to grow back prop-erly. You'll know your hair is ingrown when it causes a painful bump, which will often look red and inflamed and may be full of pus. This condition is also known as folliculitis. To help reduce the chances of developing ingrowing hairs and complications such as folliculitis:

○ Try to have a shave-free day as often as possible. Allowing the hair to grow for longer may give a better shave, which reduces the chances of problems with regrowth.

○ Be careful not to knock the top off spots that lie within the beard area. A dry shave with an electric razor may be better for this. If using a wet shave, a transparent gel will allow you to see where your razor is going.

○ If you knock the top off a spot give the skin at least an hour to recover before applying an acne cream or lotion. This will cut down on stinging or burning.

○ If using a wet shave, make sure the razor is rinsed clean with boiling water on a regular basis. This will help disinfect it and reduce the transfer of bacteria to the skin.

○ Shave in the direction of hair growth.

○ If you develop a rash of small yellow-filled spots, this is probably folliculitis. A short course of antibiotics may help. Avoid sharing towels and shaving equipment while the skin is still inflamed.

○ Use a moisturiser that contains an antibacterial agent such as Dermol® or Oilatum plus®.

○ If you can see a hair under the skin that has not pierced the surface properly, use a hot flannel as a compress to help ease the hair free. Try this for a maximum of 10 minutes, ensuring you keep the flannel as hot as possible.

○ Some men prefer to shave in the shower after the skin has been given a few minutes to warm through, avoiding the need to use a shaving gel or foam.

○ When washing, try using a lotion that contains salicylic acid. Gently rub it in small circular movements around the beard area.

Shaving tips for rosacea skin types

The secret for rosacea skin is to be as gentle as possible. Although rosacea may not appear in the beard area, the skin may still be very sensitive and need to be treated with care.

○ If wet shaving, use warm water, avoiding water that is too hot.
○ Avoid shaving products that contain alcohol.
○ For a soothing after-shave experience, try patting on aloe vera gel (as pure as possible).
○ Remember to add your sun protection after shaving.

There are plenty of things you can try to help your skin yourself. Whether you have acne or rosacea, there are many choices of product on the market. However, be cautious before parting with your money as rosacea in particular can be easily aggravated by new ingredients. It may take time for the skin to get used to new products so remember not to expect overnight miracles, and be wary of anyone who claims to offer them.

CHAPTER ELEVEN

SKIN CAMOUFLAGE AND MAKE-UP

There is nothing wrong with using camouflage and make-up to make you feel more confident and attractive. Although it is easy to consider make-up and skin camouflage to be solely for women, camouflage in particular has huge benefits for men too, so if you are a man, read on to find out how it could change your life!

Both can work wonders in hiding your acne or rosacea, making it less obvious to the naked eye. Many people actually confuse camouflage and make-up, so here are their main differences:

- **Make-up** – enhances and highlights features of the face, such as eyes and lips
- **Skin camouflage** – disguises marks on the face and can be used under make-up

Skin Camouflage

Skin camouflage is a term used to describe a range of products that are designed to conceal imperfections, scars, marks or blemishes to make them appear less obvious to the naked eye. Once applied to the skin (and as long as no soap or detergent is used) they can remain on the skin for up to three days. Camouflage used to be known as 'cosmetic camouflage', but using the term cosmetic gives the impression that it is the same as make-up used by women, which puts many people off trying it.

Camouflage creams are heavily pigmented and designed to be much more generous in their coverage than any make-up you can buy from a shop. Despite the heavy pigment, they can still be easy to apply and light in texture. Although you can choose your own green-based products from off the shelf, be aware that they will not suit all skin colours and tones. Seek help from a professional skin camouflage practitioner or a beauty counter assistant if you are not sure. The benefit of camouflage is that it will be matched to your own natural skin colour, whatever that may be. Incredibly, a selection of camouflage products is available free or for a prescription charge on the NHS, making it widely available to all.

Who is Skin Camouflage for?

Skin camouflage is suitable for any skin type or colour and even the most sensitive skins. Although some may be slightly oily in texture, there are few reports of them making acne or rosacea worse. It is sensible to suggest a patch test if you are worried. Camouflage appears to be safe on very young children. It is useful for young people, especially if the marks, scars or blemishes are causing psychological problems.

Camouflage can hide the following:

○ Healing and healed acne scars
○ Active rosacea and other skin colouring from redness through to purple or blue veins
○ Tattoos
○ Birthmarks

○ Burns
○ Pigment changes

It can be used on any part of the body, including large areas such as the back.

Where Can I Go for Camouflage Advice?

There are two choices available:

○ NHS-based services
○ Home-, clinic- or salon-based services

NHS-based services

In most parts of the UK, camouflage advice will be available from dermatology departments. Your GP can refer you to an NHS hospital-based service run by a team of volunteers who have undergone specialised training. This is known as the British Red Cross Cosmetic Camouflage, or 'Coscam', service.

The benefits of seeing a Red Cross trained practitioner are:

○ You can sometimes see them at the same time as visiting your dermatologist.
○ Some people prefer using a hospital-based service.
○ They will have been given recognised training and have a good choice of skin camouflage to offer.
○ It is a free service, although a donation to the British Red Cross is welcomed.

However, clinics may be heavily booked and appointment waiting lists can run into several weeks or possibly months. Some rural services are not offered on a regular basis and may be 'demand led', meaning they will be held only when there are enough patients to justify a volunteer's time. Ask your GP for a referral or contact your local British Red Cross branch for further information on your closest service.

Home-, clinic- or salon-based services

The alternative to waiting to see a volunteer in an NHS setting is to arrange for a consultation with someone who will charge for their time, but whose expertise will be just as high as that of a Red Cross volunteer. The advantages of these services are:

○ You can see a practitioner in the privacy of your own home, saving time and money travelling to a clinic or salon.

○ Clinic or salon-based practitioners will usually work in comfortable surroundings and will not need to spend time unpacking their camouflage kits. They may have good lighting facilities to help colour match.

○ Charges are usually very reasonable and only a one-off visit is needed.

○ The choice of camouflage creams may be wider as they will not be limited to those that can be prescribed on the NHS (the British Red Cross will often be restricted to these options).

There are currently two key providers of training in all aspects of skin camouflage: the British Association of Skin Camouflage (BASC) and the Skin Camouflage Network (SCN). Both of these organisations will have representatives who have undergone full training in every aspect of camouflage. Skin practitioners are trained to respect clients' privacy, so it is highly unlikely that a properly trained practitioner will ask awkward, probing questions about your condition. Generally, they are not there to give advice on your skin condition; indeed, most of them are not qualified to do so.

Qualified practitioners will usually have a full range of samples and will be able to offer leaflets for further sources of help and support. Whereas the British Red Cross service is free, those who work independently through the BASC or SCN will usually charge a reasonable fee for their time.

People trained in how to apply skin camouflage will encourage you to:

○ decide which colour match you feel most happy with
○ try applying the camouflage yourself
○ show you how to remove it
○ write a letter to your doctor requesting a prescription for the camouflage
○ show you tips on disguising other marks, such as freckles

CASE STUDY – JANE

I had rosacea for over 15 years before I even heard of skin camouflage. At first I thought it sounded very complicated, and something which needed a lot of skill. As somebody who has never worn make-up I thought it probably wouldn't be for me. After a while I grew increasingly fed up with my constant redness and broken veins, which were looking more noticeable with each year. In the end I thought there was probably nothing to lose so I booked an appointment with someone from the British Association of Skin Camouflage. Although I was nervous, I was also very excited about what it might look like. I arranged a time for someone to come over to my home as it meant that I was on my own ground and able to take my time.

First, the skin camouflage practitioner asked me about my skincare regime and if I would usually wear any make-up. She then showed me the different ranges of colours. I was amazed! There were far more than I had thought possible. I couldn't believe how close some of the colours seemed to be to one another. It made me realise how it might be possible to match any colour skin in the world with those!

As soon as she showed me the colours and started talking through what she was going to do, I felt that someone was now in charge and I could leave my face in her hands. I started to relax as she set to work looking at my skin in natural daylight (I sat next to the window). She seemed to be skilled at choosing the colour, going straight to one particular shade for me to start off with. Once she had put it on the back of her hand, she then gently dabbed at it and applied a little to the worst part of my cheek. She sort of patted it in rather than rubbing like you can with some creams and I was amazed by how little she had to use. After she had put it on a small area, she then used a 'fixing powder', which she then dusted off with a light brush to finish so that I didn't look too powdery. It was done in seconds!

Then she handed me her mirror. I really could not believe that, for the first time in years, my skin seemed 'normal' in that area. I must admit that it brought a tear to my eye, and before I knew it, we were both shedding a little tear!

She talked me through removing it and encouraged me to try for myself. From start to finish, I think it took just over five minutes. She then told me that she would write a letter for me to give to my doctor explaining what she had done and would include details of the make and colour of the camouflage. A couple of days later this arrived and I took it to my doctor who then prescribed me the camouflage.

I know it hasn't cured my rosacea, but it has made it disappear to the outside world and I have immense confidence now. It really was a painless, enjoyable and illuminating experience and I would recommend it for anyone – even men!

Make-up

Once camouflage has been applied, make-up can be used on top. If you have little or no confidence in using it, you might find it helpful to book a make-up lesson. You can get good advice on make-up from the following people:

A professional make-up artist

You can find contact details for make-up artists in telephone and online directories and wedding magazines. Make-up artists may be based in a skin clinic and double up as beauty therapists. You can ask them questions as they make you up, teasing out some of their top tips. If you have already been matched for skin camouflage (see pages 216–20) then take that along with you and ask them to work with it. They may be able to visit you in your own home, and usually one visit or consultation should be all you need. A good make-up artist should ensure that you are confident in applying your own make-up. There will be a charge for this service and prices vary according to experience and location.

Beauty and make-up counter staff

This may be a bit more 'hit and miss' as, inevitably, they will be trying to sell you products and you'll no doubt be treated to the sales patter. They are free, however, and will often be able to:

○ offer advice on make-up and different 'looks' you may want to achieve
○ show you how to apply make-up
○ give you a set time if you make an appointment in advance

However, be aware that they are usually based in a public space, so others may be able to see you and may even stop and watch. If you use skin camouflage, apply it before you visit the beauty counter.

Although such services are free, staff may be working on commission and have an extra incentive to sell. Don't commit to buying anything if you are unsure. This might mean leaving the store or clinic to give yourself a chance to assess how well your make-up is staying on and how good the colours are in natural daylight. Ask the counter staff to write down all the products you have tried so you will know what to buy if you are satisfied.

Types of make-up to conceal your acne or rosacea

Make-up comes in hundreds of colours and a wide choice of formats. The range seems endless, from traditional powders, liquids, blocks and creams, to the latest technology using sprays or cream-to-powder. This section will explore some of these options. It will focus on the choice of foundation make-up used on the face to conceal rather than make-up used to enhance, which is what eye and lip make-up is designed to do.

Mineral make-up

This is the latest in make-up for any skin type, and the range seems to grow every day. Mineral make-up is made from finely ground minerals and can be applied using a large, soft brush in a light circular motion. It is also available in liquid formulations which are applied by hand or by brush. It claims to reflect light from the face to avoid the skin looking 'flat' and toneless, which can happen with some heavier make-ups.

They claim to have a number of major advantages over traditional foundations:

○ They are fragrance free so ideal for those with sensitivities to fragrances or perfumes.

○ They contain a sun protection factor (SPF) of 15 to help protect the skin from the sun.

○ They have anti-inflammatory properties, helping to control breakouts of spots or irritation.

○ The powders don't leave a powdery residue on the skin.

○ There is a wide choice of colours.

○ Ease of application means they don't leave a 'tide mark' on outer edges of the face.

A word of caution: apply it a layer at a time to avoid over-loading, which may leave the face looking slightly over made-up. The powder formulation may need to be applied by shaking a little into the lid and dipping the brush into that rather than collecting a lump on the brush.

Cover sticks and concealers

There is no real difference between a cover stick and a concealer; both have the ultimate aim of covering a mark to reduce its appearance, making it less obvious. Consider this to be a mini 'camouflage' product. It can be dabbed directly onto individual spots or dabbed on and spread to cover wider areas of redness. Like skin camouflage, concealers and cover sticks can also be ideal for men's skin.

Cover sticks and concealers are available in different consistencies. The usual rule is the thicker the consistency, the longer it will last. The downside to this is that thicker consistencies can look less natural, so apply them sparingly. Take the time to find one that suits your skin tone exactly, rather than selecting a standard green tint off the shelf. The extra time and effort will make the difference between it working well or looking too obvious. Green tint sticks or pots can, however, be very useful to hide redness.

TOP CONCEALER AND COVER STICK ADVICE

○ Choose the right shade for you. Match the colour to your skin in strong daylight to get the best results.

○ Some will have an extra spot-fighting ingredient such as salicylic acid or tea tree oil, which can help heal an inflamed spot. However, these may not be ideal for people with sensitive skin, particularly rosacea. If you have rosacea, seek skin soothing or extra gentle concealers.

○ Avoid applying too much. Start off with the least amount possible and build up coverage if it is still necessary. Keep checking in good, natural daylight.

○ Keep direct skin contact to a minimum to avoid the cover stick or concealer becoming a breeding ground for bacteria.

○ Once it has been applied to the skin, use fingers, brush or an applicator sponge to gently blend it in.

○ Normal foundation can be applied on top of the concealer.

CHAPTER TWELVE
SUN PROTECTION

As the sun doesn't shine every day of the year in Britain, many people run open-armed into the first rays that follow a long, dark, damp winter or a soggy spring. It's natural to enjoy the warmth of the sun and the feel-good factor it gives. However, with the rise in skin cancer, we can no longer afford to be a nation of sun-lovers who deny the risks of unprotected sun exposure. Rosacea and acne skin types have their own needs when it comes to sun protection, and a few key principles apply to both. It needn't be all doom and gloom, though; being sensible about sun exposure and under-standing the risks of long-term damage can help to ensure that being sun-wise doesn't necessarily mean being totally sun-shy.

Many people with acne or rosacea have some long-held beliefs about the sun and its relationship to their skin problems. Let's consider these in more detail.

Rosacea Skin and Exposure to Sunlight

Many people with rosacea believe they should avoid any type of sun exposure because of the risk of worsening the symptoms. However, the skin can gain some goodness from sunlight, including vitamin D, which plays a vital role in helping the body to build and maintain strong teeth and bones. We usually get all the vitamin D we need during 'normal' exposure to sunlight.

As rosacea mainly affects older people, any substantial reduction in exposure to sunlight needs to be balanced with finding other sources of vitamin D. A very small amount of sun exposure with adequate sun protection can still help maintain some vitamin D production and is worth considering. However, if your skin type is very sensitive to sunlight and you need to avoid it at all costs, then consider a diet rich in vitamin D. Good sources include fatty fish, such as herring and tuna, and eggs. If you are a vegan, try vegetable margarines or soya milk. The maximum recommended daily allowance for this vitamin is 10 micrograms, a very small amount.

Rosacea-friendly sun protection

Recommending protection for this skin type is challenging as people with rosacea have such a wide variety of needs. Mineral make-up has many fans because it conceals while it protects from the sun at SPF 15. However, this is not usually suitable for men. The Australian sun cream experts, Sunsense™, have a wide range of products that are highly recommended by people with rosacea. The Daily Face is a strong favourite.

Acne Skin and Exposure to Sunlight

For many years, some people have firmly believed that sunlight has 'cured' their acne problems. A short break in the sun that offered a miracle cure is frequently followed by regular trips to a tanning salon to help maintain the improvement. It's understandable to feel elation at seeing the skin improved, and a tan may, for some people, give the impression of good health. This may be further supported by people proclaiming how 'healthy' and 'well' someone looks after a holiday. This is natural. However,

HOW TO PROTECT ROSACEA SKIN FROM THE SUN

○ Minimise exposure to sunlight.

○ If staying out of the sun, remember to keep vitamin D levels up either by diet or by supplements.

○ Keep the sun protection factor (SPF) as high as possible (SPF 30+ is recommended).

○ Reapply sunscreen every two hours.

○ Look for sun protection creams/lotions/gels designed for sensitive skin types.

○ If your skin is particularly sensitive, keep a handy container of your favourite sun protection in your bag or in the car, together with a pack of hand wipes, and apply whenever needed.

○ Keep the skin cool with water sprays and fans. Try a homemade face spritzer – mix two drops of lavender oil into pre-boiled and cooled water and use a plant spray bottle to cool the face whenever needed (avoiding the eyes).

○ Wear a wide-brimmed hat.

○ Remember to wear a good quality pair of sunglasses that fully cover the eye area, especially if you have rosacea-linked problems with your eyes.

○ If your eyes are sensitive to sunlight, soak some cotton wool pads in fresh water and wrap in a sealed bag. Keep it in the fridge and transfer to a cool bag just before going out. This cooling homemade eye patch will relieve most sensitive eyes.

○ Check medicines to ensure they don't cause sun sensitivity. If they do, take maximum protection measures including using a full sunblock, wearing a hat and keeping to shaded areas.

the reason for this is not necessarily to do with the acne fading but with how rested we may feel and how a tan gives a deceptive image of looking healthy. It is, ironically, damage to the skin that makes us appear so healthy.

When skin is exposed to UV light, the melanocytes located in the dermis (the second layer of skin) produce a colour pigment designed to help protect the skin. This is either brown or, in the case of fairer skin types, reddish, giving the appearance of a tan. The tan will help conceal any minor visible discolouration, such as redness or blotches, kill the acne-making bacteria *P. acnes* and reduce oiliness. However, the benefits are short-lived as the skin will return to its original condition, with extra damage due to UV exposure, soon after exposure to UV is withdrawn.

Some people claim their acne gets worse in the sun, with a type of acne called 'acne Majorca' named after this very condition. In addition, sweating can make acne worse. This, together with the combination of heat and some oily sun creams, can greatly worsen the problem.

Danger: using sun beds to treat acne

Sun beds are increasingly frowned upon. No dermatologist is likely to support the use of UV beds unless under strict medical supervision. The amount of UV you are exposed to may damage the skin, greatly increasing your chance of developing skin moles and changes that can easily lead to skin cancers — sunbeds double the risk of skin cancer. People who have used sun beds over a long period can have skin that appears leathery and old before its time. Evidence is mounting on the dangers of sun beds, and their use is likely to be further restricted in the future.

UV light does not treat acne, it just disguises spots. With such a wide choice of alternative ways of safely treating acne, this should be firmly crossed off the list of options unless you are prepared to take such risks for a temporary benefit.

Acne-friendly sun protection

One of the key enemies of acne is oil. Many sun creams, gels, lotions or sprays will inevitably contain oil, so choose with caution. Look for those that are labelled 'non-comedogenic' or 'oil-free'.

Some brands which are highly recommended for acne skins are from ranges that also give very high protection. Two manufacturers regularly recommended by people with acne-prone skin include Sunsense™ and Neutrogena®. Many also recommend mineral make-up, which automatically gives a protection SPF of 15 without causing blocked pores or oiliness.

Understanding UV Radiation

Each skin type will have its own needs when it comes to sun protection. Understanding the fundamentals about ultraviolet (UV) radiation – what it is and what it does to us – is the first step in getting protection right.

Ultraviolet rays can be split into the following groups:

○ UVA: These damage the elastin and collagen fibres supporting the skin – signs of aging are the most common results, thus the 'A' could stand for aging. UVA penetrates deeper into the skin than UVB.
○ UVB: These rays are responsible for burning and tanning the skin, so 'B' could stand for burning. We may think a suntan makes us look bronzed and healthy but the darkening of skin pigment is just nature's way of protecting our skin.

○ UVC: This type of UV radiation can cause the greatest damage but it should be filtered out by the earth's ozone layer.

All surfaces either absorb UV or reflect it back. Sun is reflected off light surfaces such as snow and sand but is absorbed better on darker surfaces and behind glass.

What is an SPF?

SPF stands for sun protection factor. It is a rough guide to how long skin can be exposed to solar energy before it reddens (which is the first sign of damage). Therefore, if you usually burn within 15 minutes without sun protection (this will probably be skin types 1 and 2), then you can calculate the total time you can stay exposed if you use an SPF of 15:

○ 15 minutes before normally turning red x SPF 15 gives 15 times the usual amount of time before normally turning red = 3 hours 45 minutes' protection

Another example:
If the skin turns red after 20 minutes and you use an SPF of 30 this would mean:

○ 20 minutes before normally turning red x SPF 30 gives 30 times the usual amount of time before normally turning red = 10 hours' protection

Calculating the amount of UV you are exposed to depends on:

○ The amount of time you spend in the sun

○ The time of day: the midday sun will be far stronger than the evening or early morning sun

○ Where you are: the closer to the equator, the stronger the sunlight

○ If exposed to full or partial sun: seeking shady areas will still give some degree of exposure, but it will be greatly reduced. You should still use sun protection in the shade.

The protection you gain from your sunscreen will depend upon:

○ Your skin type (see the Fitzpatrick scale, page 119). The paler your type, the more easily you will burn

○ How much sunscreen is applied and if it is applied properly: any gaps will leave the skin exposed to dangerous burning

○ Any activities you undertake. Swimming, sweating or friction such as rolling in sand is likely to remove sunscreen. Reapply as soon as possible

The SPF rating applies only to protection to UVB radiation. However, there are moves to give useful information regarding UVA protection on all sunscreens.

Applying Sunscreen

Traditionally, sunscreen is applied the moment the skin is exposed to sunlight. Some scientists argue this is already too late. In order to give the skin enough time to absorb the sunscreen it should be applied 15–30 minutes *before* going outside and then again approximately 30 minutes after first exposure. Any further applications may not be needed unless you have gone swimming or have rubbed it off. However, other scientists argue that applying a sunscreen every two hours will give maximum protection.

Follow this guide to get the best benefit from your sunscreen:

- ○ Apply evenly with an equal thickness to all areas. How much to use is difficult to quantify as larger people have more skin than smaller people, so it can only be estimated. However, average faces might need up to a quarter or a third of a teaspoon of sun cream.
- ○ When applying the sunscreen to the face remember to cover all areas that are exposed. That includes any exposed skin on the ears or top of the head and neck for those who don't have hair coverage. These areas will require extra sunscreen after the allowance for the face has been used.
- ○ If using any acne or rosacea creams, lotions or gels, apply at least 15 minutes before the first application of sunscreen to allow them to be absorbed properly.
- ○ Check if your medication is likely to make skin more sensitive to sun exposure. Read the patient information leaflet that comes with your medicine or ask your GP or pharmacist. If the leaflet recommends avoiding sun exposure, or describes 'photosensitivity' as a common side-effect, then use the maximum sun protection possible and keep the face shaded beneath a wide-brimmed hat.

If you are worried that your skin may react to a new sun cream, carry out a patch test on an area usually affected by your skin problem. Patch testing on your arm or leg may not have the same effect as trying it on the face.

Physical sunscreens (sunblocks)

These block or reflect the sun's rays. They include:

○ Hats, clothing, sun umbrellas
○ Opaque products containing titanium dioxide and micro-nised titanium dioxide, similar to those worn by Australian cricketers and lifeguards. These total sunblocks can also block pores, trapping oil beneath, so use with caution in acne skin types

Chemical sunscreens

Sunscreens use chemicals to absorb ultraviolet light. The most common of the absorption chemicals is PABA (para-aminobenzoic acid), which absorbs UVB. However, PABA may cause irritation or an allergic reaction in those with sensitive skin. Patch test it first if you are not sure.

Other sunscreen chemicals include:

○ Anthranilates: absorb UVA and UVB
○ Benzophenones: absorb UVA
○ Cinnamates: absorb UVB
○ Ecamsules: absorb UVA

Ideally you will use a sunscreen that can absorb both UVA and UVB.

With even the most sensitive of skins, it is not necessary to lock yourself away. The benefits gained from even a small amount of UV exposure are worth considering as long as you take necessary precautions to avoid overheating or burning. Using the right sun protection doesn't need to cost a fortune.

EXTREMELY SUN-SENSITIVE SKIN

Some people find it impossible to tolerate any sunlight at all on their skin, reporting an unbearable sensation of burning or tingling. If these sound like your symptoms, visit your GP to make sure it is not another condition called polymorphic light eruption (PLE). PLE signs and symptoms include:

○ Feeling of skin burning, sometimes even through light clothing and windows

○ A slight delay of a few hours or days before a red, spotty rash is seen, which can last up to 10 days on exposed areas

○ More common in women than men

○ It differs to prickly heat by appearing on any area exposed to the sun (prickly heat usually occurs on the body where clothing can irritate it and is a result of over-heating)

Whatever the diagnosis, this type of skin can be effectively helped by wearing light-coloured clothing to reflect light, avoiding going out during the hottest part of the day and by using a total sunblock everyday.

If sunlight feels like it is burning the skin through windows, purchase a roll of UV protection film. This is transparent, easy to fit and effective. Stockists can be found on the internet. However, glass is a very good natural filter of UV light, although it doesn't filter out 100 per cent of UV radiation.

CHAPTER THIRTEEN
FEELING GOOD ABOUT YOURSELF

Having acne or rosacea can be about far more than just a red face or inflamed, angry spots. For some people the experience of having a skin problem can leave them feeling any or all of the following:

- Desperate
- Alone
- Depressed
- Suicidal
- Confused
- Embarrassed
- Ashamed
- Distressed

It's understandable to experience these feelings if you don't know what to do or feel frustrated because nobody seems to care. The key to overcoming such feelings is to recognise them, acknowledge them and then seek appropriate help for them while also treating the skin. If the skin is successfully treated, most people find any connected feelings of depression will improve quite quickly. However, some depression may also have links to other issues unrelated to the condition of the skin, or may need more than just an improvement in the acne or rosacea to disappear. Many websites, patient support groups and health professionals can offer fantastic help with the symptoms of depression and are well worth consulting for signposting to other services if necessary.

Some studies suggest that young people with acne are 15 times more likely to be depressed enough to feel suicidal, compared with young people without acne.[1] You don't have to feel suicidal, though, to be classified as being depressed. Some small changes with how you feel can have a long-term impact on your mental health. Half of the battle with depression is being able to recognise you have it in order to take the first steps to seeking help.

A study of the psychosocial impact of rosacea found that this condition can leave people experiencing difficulty functioning in everyday life. They have a worse general health perception as well as a higher level of anxiety and depression, compared with a group of people without rosacea.[2]

Signs of Depression

What is depression and how can we know the difference between feeling 'a bit down' and being depressed? Feelings of depression can vary from mild to severe and may change from day to day. To be fairly measured, depression should be rated over a period of time, for example comparing how you feel now to last month. If you are feeling 'a bit down', is that the same as feeling like you want to take your own life? Other signs of depression can include:

- Loss of appetite or excessive eating
- Feeling lethargic and uninterested in doing anything new
- A change in usual behaviour, such as erratic mood swings

○ Being unable to sleep
○ Crying for no apparent reason
○ Feelings of unworthiness

There are a variety of quizzes, questionnaires and self-completed tests designed to help test and measure depression. One example of a questionnaire specifically for those with acne is called the assessment of the psychological and social effects of acne (APSEA).

Assessment of the psychological and social effects of acne

This is an example of a section of questions posed in the brief questionnaire. While it is not a tool for diagnosis, it can be helpful to give an idea of how acne is affecting confidence and wellbeing. The higher the score, the worse the problem may be considered to be. Those with the highest results are normally considered to be the most urgent to treat.

Read the following carefully and circle the number that most accurately represents how you feel.

How has your skin condition limited the following activities or made them more difficult or awkward, or less enjoyable, since you have had acne?

Going shopping
Never   0   1   2   3   4   5   6   7   8   9   10   All the time

Going out socially to meet friends
Never   0   1   2   3   4   5   6   7   8   9   10   All the time

Going away for weekends, holidays and outings
Never   0   1   2   3   4   5   6   7   8   9   10   All the time

Eating out

Never 0 1 2 3 4 5 6 7 8 9 10 All the time

Using public changing rooms/swimming pools

Never 0 1 2 3 4 5 6 7 8 9 10 All the time

Do you think your appearance will interfere with your chances of future employment?

Strongly 0 1 2 3 4 5 6 7 8 9 10 Strongly
disagree   agree

This set of questions could easily be applied to those with rosacea. It may help to use this self-assessment tool when visiting your GP, dermatologist or nurse about your skin.

Many factors other than acne can contribute towards depression, but regardless of the cause, depression must be recognised and managed early. If you think you may be depressed, or if someone you care about has any of the above symptoms, contact your doctor for help. Many websites provide helpful guidance for anyone affected by depression, and treatments can make a huge difference to general mood and outlook.

Picking up the signs of depression in young people with acne

It is quite unlikely that a teenager with acne will feel comfortable enough to ask outright for help, so it will be left to worried parents, friends, teachers or doctors/nurses to take the opportunity to raise the subject in a tactful, helpful manner. When I was running the Acne Support Group helpline, many calls were from mothers of 16-year-old boys. This seemed to be a particularly difficult age for parents to communicate with their children, and vice versa. Boys at this age are likely to be under growing pressures such as taking exams, peer pressure and sexual awareness, which may link closely to their feelings of confidence. At this complicated time of life, having acne is bound to knock confidence. It may lead to a variety of behaviours including retreating to the bedroom, skipping school, avoiding sports or social events and poor exam results.

If you are watching someone change in front of your eyes from a confident, happy person to a withdrawn, moody individual, how can you be certain it is not just the typical signs of teenage angst? Some verbal clues may help point towards depression, including statements such as:

○ 'I'm better off dead.'
○ 'You'd be better off without me.'
○ 'What's the point?

It is also possible that a person feeling like this won't say these things to others, but may have internal 'conversations' (common to us all, every day) in their heads. The only clues to the outside world might be a change in character and physically looking defeated, miserable, sad or withdrawn.

Visual clues of depression may include:

○ Not bothering to get dressed
○ Not bothering to wash
○ Wearing dirty clothes
○ Not bothering with hair or make-up

More obvious clues will be avoiding eye contact and keeping the face covered as much as possible. The key is to look for changes in 'normal' behaviour.

Helping Someone who May be Depressed

Sometimes it may be very hard to raise the subject of depression with someone who has chosen to lock themselves away or who stays silent and sullen in your presence. Suddenly saying 'I think you are depressed' may not be the approach that works for everyone, although much may be gained by being straightforward for some. If you find it too hard to know what to say, then try writing a letter or note to that person and leave it somewhere you know they will see it. Writing allows you to express your concern, and reading it allows the person to take stock of your worries without slamming a door in your face or shouting back. If you feel this might be a good way of putting your worries to the person, start by explaining how much you care about them and how worried you are. No matter what that person may think of you writing them a letter, they will be left in no doubt about your motives for helping them.

Dealing with suicidal feelings

If you or someone you know feels so unhappy, helpless or desperate that they want to take their own life, call the Samaritans on 08457 90 90 90 or your family doctor immediately. Feeling an impulse to take your own life may be strong, but will often pass. Seek the help you feel you need immediately.

Dysmorphophobic Acne

This is a condition (pronounced *dis-more-for-fobik*) where someone with mild to completely absent acne suffers from a disturbed (or distorted) body image. Even in the absence of typical acne lesions, they consider they have severe acne and may suffer many of the psychological and social symptoms described above.

Some doctors are reluctant to treat acne that is barely visible and it may take a lot of convincing for a person to be referred to an NHS dermatologist. People are sometimes prepared to spend up to several thousand pounds of their own money on consultations, treatments and even surgery that may be unnecessary. Some dermatologists may choose to treat this type of mild but psychologically affecting acne with the strongest treatment currently available (isotretinoin, see pages 74–82). However, it is vital to ensure that the underlying psychological problems are not ignored and to seek help from a professional able to recognise and treat this condition.

Some of the symptoms of dysmorphophobia include:

○ Excessive mirror checking
○ Worrying or obsessively thinking about appearance (this can be for several hours a day)
○ Believing they have severe acne when others are unable to see anything, or can see very little

As a person's obsession with their skin increases, it will often affect their interaction with other people socially, at work or at school. Keeping a skin diary (see pages 193–5) or just noting thoughts and actions related to this condition may help a person become aware of their, often destructive, behaviour. Professional help, using either cognitive behaviour therapy (CBT), counselling or a psychologist, is usually very beneficial.

CONCLUSION

While it might be argued that acne is a rite of passage, or that a red face a normal part of 'getting older', there should be no reason for anyone to feel they simply have to 'put up' with their symptoms. No one should be willing to wait to grow out of their condition without the knowledge of the wide range of treatment options open to them. Nor should ignorance from a doctor, nurse or pharmacist mean acne or rosacea has to be left untreated or poorly managed. Scarring from acne can be a permanent reminder of what is usually a temporary problem, and most scars occur when acne is not properly managed. However, there are many well-trained healthcare professionals willing and able to help. In addition, this book has acknowledged the perseverance and patience required to stick to treatments that may take time to work. Impatience is the enemy of acne and rosacea!

I hope this book will also help parents to support children with acne. We cannot force someone to use or try treatments that we believe are best for them, but as parents we can give our children the relevant information and then step back and allow them to make these choices for themselves.

This book has acknowledged the common frustrations felt by thousands with rosacea. It has attempted to unravel the maze of theories surrounding this still largely mysterious condition.

Rosacea is not a simple disease; it is a combination of many symptoms ranging from the mild to the severe. It requires a close examination of lifestyle and everyday living environments, which can be tiresome and tedious. However, the rewards for discovering your own triggers will be huge; knowing what to avoid can give you back a sense of liberation and, most importantly, control.

Nobody needs to be at the mercy of their skin. No matter how bad your condition there is always something you can take, use or try that will help. I hope this book will be the companion you need to help you find the answers. Good luck and stay patient!

GLOSSARY

Acne conglobata a highly inflammatory form of acne that has a variety of comedones, nodules and abscesses.

Acne fulminans an aggressive type of acne that may also cause joint aches and pains. It is associated with a problem with the immune system and can be very hard to treat successfully.

Acne Majorca a type of acne associated with the use of oily sun lotions and creams, in combination with consistently high temperatures and humid conditions. It is also known as acne aestivalis.

Acne mechanica acne resulting from anything that traps heat against the body for a prolonged period of time, or rubs or puts pressure onto the skin.

Acne vulgaris the common acne experienced by most people.

Acupressure a blend of acupuncture and pressure where the hands are used to help relieve a variety of conditions. It works on the theory of stimulating the meridian system, which is responsible for rebalancing a person's 'life force'.

Acupuncture very fine needles are inserted at various points around the body to help relieve a variety of symptoms. This originates from China and has been used for thousands of years.

Adapalene the name given to a retinoid gel or cream used to treat mild–moderate acne.

Alternative therapy the name given to any type of healing practice which is not considered to be 'conventional', i.e. proven to work and can be prescribed by medical doctors. Alternative therapies cover a broad range of options including traditional Chinese medicine, aromatherapy, meditation, yoga, etc. If they are used alone as a treatment they are alternative, but if they are used alongside conventional treatments they are considered 'complementary'.

Antimicrobial includes anything which has the action of killing or preventing any type of microorganisms and includes antibiotics, antivirals and antifungals. They can be used to kill a variety of organisms either on the body or on non-living objects such as disinfectants used on work surfaces.

Aromatherapy a form of alternative therapy using essential oils extracted from a variety of plants. They can be inhaled or rubbed into the skin. It is believed they work in two different ways: by the aroma affecting the brain (stimulating 'feel-good' emotions) and by their effect directly on the area applied, either through the action of rubbing or by their own healing powers.

Atrophic scars any type of scar where there is a loss of tissue, giving the appearance of a 'dip' or 'pitting'. This includes box-car and ice-pick scarring.

Ayurvedic translates from the Sanskrit word meaning 'the science of life' and describes a variety of traditional Indian medicines. It is a type of alternative medicine and its philosophy is to prevent disease and promote healthy living by using the mind and body together, rather than just treating a condition or disease alone.

Blackhead also referred to as an 'open comedone', this is the result of the build-up of excess oil in the sebaceous gland. It appears as a slightly raised black dot on the skin.

Chinese herbal medicine also known as traditional Chinese medicine (TCM), this is a range of medicines and practices that originate in China and are used to treat a variety of conditions. They are considered to be a type of alternative medicine. Examples of TCM include acupuncture, Shiatsu massage and the preparation of specially made herbal teas.

Comedone the word to describe a solid blockage in the skin. A comedone can be either a 'whitehead' (a closed comedone) or a 'blackhead' (an open comedone). These are the non-inflammatory type of acne.

Complementary therapy a term used to describe a variety of treatments and procedures that are used at the same time as taking modern 'conventional' medicines. Complementary therapies include treatments and methods with ancient roots, such as Indian (Ayurvedic) and Chinese medicines (traditional Chinese medicine), as well as a range of relaxation techniques, such as meditation, yoga and massages.

Corticosteroids any type of medication that contains steroids. These are a type of hormone commonly used to reduce inflammation. They are available in a variety of different forms including tablets, sprays, inhalers and injections.

Cyst a membrane-covered growth. It can be formed on the surface of an organ and they are either filled with air, infected fluids or semi-solid substances such as sebum.

Dermatologist a doctor qualified in dermatology (the study of skin diseases). In the UK there are approximately 2,000 dermatologists. As well as studying the skin, they are also trained in diseases and conditions affecting the nails, hair and scalp.

Dissecting cellulitis of the scalp also called perifolliculitis capitis abscedens et suffodiens. A chronic (long-lasting) scalp disorder involving inflamed nodules and redness of the scalp. Its causes are unknown and it is difficult to treat effectively.

Dysmorphophobic acne a person's apparent obsession and pre-occupation with an imagined defect (in this case acne). It may incorporate an excessive fear of judgement by others and may lead to social seclusion and may be accompanied by other 'nervous' disorders such as anorexia nervosa, bulimia nervosa, compulsive overeating or obsessive compulsive disorder (OCD).

Epidermis this is the outer layer of the skin, composed of four or five layers (depending on the part of the body). This is where skin cells are shed.

Erythematotelangiectatic rosacea this is identified by the appearance of flushing and persistent redness to the central face area. Broken veins may or may not be present. This type of rosacea can also cause other symptoms such as stinging, swelling or blurring.

Follicle a small spherical group of cells that form a cavity. In the skin, this follicle is where the hair, sweat and grease are produced.

Folliculitis inflammation of the hair follicles usually caused by the bacteria known as *Bacterium Staphylococcus*. It tends to be more common in humid conditions where clothing may trap sweat, making it an ideal breeding ground for bacteria.

Herbal medicine this may also be known as herbalism. It is the use of medicines based upon plants and plant extracts and will usually be given by an alternative or complementary practitioner. The most well-known type of herbal medicines are those given in Chinese medicines, but many other types exist such as Ayurvedic, Tibetan and Kampo.

Hidradenitis suppurativa a skin disease with three key symptoms: 1. deep-seated nodules; 2. location will usually be in the apocrine gland areas in the armpits, groin, breast and buttocks and 3. will be chronic in nature, meaning it may heal but will often re-occur. It is believed there may be a genetic link.

Homeopathy a type of holistic therapy that uses highly diluted preparations, based on the belief of treating 'like with like,' i.e. using a substance that would normally *cause* the symptoms.

Hypertrophic scar a type of scar that is raised above the normal level of the skin. It may be red and itchy, eventually fading to become flat and pale in some cases.

Hypnotherapy any type of therapy that puts a patient into a hypnotic state of deep relaxation. It uses suggestive language to direct the unconscious mind to help the body to heal.

Inflammatory acne these spots are filled with bacteria that cause the inflammatory response of redness, swelling and tenderness. They may or may not contain pus.

Keloid scar a type of raised scar that contains collagen. It is caused as a result of an overgrowth of granulation tissue at the site of an injury (such as a spot). It feels firm and rubbery to the touch and can be flesh-coloured, red or dark brown in colour. Unlike hypertrophic scarring, this type of scar will commonly grow beyond the area of the original injury and may spread to a much larger site.

Laser therapy laser stands for light amplification by stimulated emission of radiation. It is a mechanism for emitting electromagnetic radiation. Lasers are used medically either to cut, burn or destroy tissue. Laser beams are so precise they can be used safely on small areas of the body without damaging surrounding healthy tissue.

Lesion in dermatology the word used to broadly describe any type of spot. It can be roughly translated from the Latin word *laesio* which means injury.

Light therapy also known as phototherapy, this uses specific waves of light to stimulate the skin's healing response. Light therapy used to treat acne and rosacea will usually be set at the visible violet light (seen as blue light), which targets bacteria, in combination with red light, which triggers the skin to become rejuvenated.

Macule this is commonly used to describe a healing spot which is neither raised nor pitted in appearance. It comes from the Latin word *macula*, meaning spot or blemish.

Melanin the substance that gives skin and hair its colouring. Melanin is produced by cells called melanocytes. It provides a natural protection from sunlight. The more melanin produced, the darker the skin will appear.

Microcomedone tiny blockages in the skin which are usually invisible to the naked eye. These are considered to be the beginning stage of all spots and are caused by a plug of oil and dead skin cells.

Naturopathy a holistic approach to the general health, diet and lifestyle of a person through the belief in healing using natural remedies and practices in harmony. It is considered to be one of many alternative types of remedy and may include a range of healing practices such as acupuncture, ozone therapy or colonic hydrotherapy.

Neuropathic rosacea bouts of burning and pain in the central facial area. These bouts will usually last longer than 30 minutes.

Nicotinamide a form of vitamin B3 which is used in anti-inflammatory acne medication.

Nodular cystic acne a variety of severe acne in which the skin has both nodules (deep, hard red lumps) and cysts (soft, large fluid-filled spots).

Non-inflammatory acne any type of acne in which there is no redness or inflammation. This is commonly seen in both open and closed comedones.

Non-transient erythema persistent redness of the skin most commonly seen in rosacea.

Ocular rosacea a variety of rosacea symptoms that affect the eye. These may include redness, grittiness, swollen or inflamed eyelids, watering or itching.

Papule a red type of spot which appears as a small bump. They are usually less than 1 cm in diameter and are an inflamed type of acne.

Papulopustular rosacea the usual symptoms are central facial redness with papules or pustules. This type is most likely to resemble common acne, but no comedones will be present.

Phymatous rosacea areas of skin thickening that eventually cause enlargement. The most common site for this is on the nose, although it can also occur on the chin, cheeks, forehead and ears.

Pigmentation marks skin discolouration after a spot has healed. These are either pink, darker than the normal skin colour (hyperpigmentation) or lacking colour (hypopigmentation).

Polycystic ovary syndrome (PCOS) a condition where the ovaries contain many small cysts, usually no bigger than 8 mm in size. Classic signs include acne, irregular periods, male-pattern hair growth and weight gain.

Post-acne hyperpigmentation the name given to dark marks left behind after a spot has healed. It is caused by the skin producing too much melanin.

Propionibacterium acnes (*P. acnes*) the name of the bacterium that is present in the skin that causes the typical inflammatory spots such as papules and pustules. It is an anaerobic bacterium, meaning it thrives in oxygenless environments that are created in a blocked hair follicle.

Pustule a pus-filled inflamed spot that contains dead skin cells and bacteria. It will appear with a yellow-coloured head and may be surrounded by an area of redness.

Qi the 'energy flow' of the body. The concept is used in many alternative therapies, especially Chinese, Japanese and Indian.

Reflexology a method of applying pressure using the thumb or finger on areas of the foot. It is a form of alternative therapy that aims to identify areas of the body 'mapped' on the sole of the foot to help give a diagnosis of condition and to help heal by gentle manipulation.

Rolling scars a type of scarring that is tethered to tissue beneath the skin, making it appear to 'ruckle'. To be treated successfully, the tethered tissue beneath the skin needs to be released using a fine needle or scalpel.

Sebaceous gland microscopic glands that produce an oil called sebum. They are found in the greatest abundance on the face and scalp and are almost totally absent on the soles of the feet and palms of the hand. The sebaceous gland makes up part of the pilosebaceous unit that also consists of the hair, hair follicle and arrector pili muscle.

Sebum the waxy oil produced within the sebaceous gland. It is believed it acts to protect and keep skin and hair waterproof, although it is also argued that it actually serves no useful purpose.

Skin camouflage the name given to a range of heavily pigmented (coloured) cosmetics used specifically to conceal and camouflage a range of skin marks, scars or discolouration.

Telangiectasia red, dilated or broken superficial blood vessels on the surface of the skin. They are also known as spider veins.

Topical antibiotics a range of antibiotic treatments that are applied directly to the skin. Topical means 'locally'.

Topical retinoids a range of retinoid treatments that are applied directly to the skin.

Transient erythema short-lasting redness.

Whitehead a type of non-inflammatory acne in which the skin appears to have a pale or skin-coloured bump. This is also known as a closed comedone and is the result of a blockage further down the sebaceous gland that has slightly raised the skin's surface.

REFERENCES

Chapter 1

1   James, William D. 'Acne', *New England Journal of Medicine*, 352: 1463–1472, April 7 2005

2   Bell, M.A. 'A comparative study of the ultrastructure of the sebaceous glands in man and other primates', *Journal of Investigative Dermatology*, 62: 132, 1974

3   Blake, J., Holland, K.T. and Cunliffe, W.J. 'The development and regression of individual acne lesions', *Journal of Investigative Dermatology*, 87: 130, 1986

4   Collier, C., Harper, J., Cantrell, W., Wang, W., Foster, K. and Elewski, B. 'The prevalence of acne in adults 20 years and older', *Journal of the American Academy of Dermatology:* 58: 56–9, January 2008

5, 6   Smithard, A., Glazebrook, C. and Williams, H.C. 'Acne prevalence, knowledge about acne and psychological morbidity in mid-adolescence: a community-based study', *British Journal of Dermatology*, 145(2): 274–9, August 2001

7   Carmina, Enrico and Lobo, Rogerio A. 'Polycystic ovary syndrome (PCOS)', *Journal of Clinical Endocrinology and Metabolism*, 84(6), 1897–9, 1999

Chapter 2

1   Cordain, L., Lindeberg, S., Hurtado, M., Hill, K., Eaton, S.B., Brand-Miller, J. 'Acne vulgaris: a disease of Western civilization', *Archives of Dermatology* 138(12): 1584–90, December 2002

2   Capitano, B., Sinagra, J.L., Ottaviani, M., Bordignon, V., Amantea, A.

and Picardo, M. 'Smokers' acne: a new clinical entity?', *British Journal of Dermatology*, 157(5): 1070–1, 2007

3   Tan, J.K., Vasey, K. and Fung, K.Y. 'Beliefs and perceptions of patients with acne', *Journal of the American Academy of Dermatology*, 44: 439–45, 2001

4   Cunliffe, W.J., Gould, D.J., 'Prevalence of facial acne vulgaris in late adolescence and in young adults', *British Medical Journal*, 1: 1109–10, 1979

Chapter 3

1. Toyoda, M., Morohashi, M. 'An overview of topical antibiotics for acne treatment', *Dermatology* 196: 130–4, 1998

2. Eady E.A., Jones C.E., Tipper J.L., et al. 'Antibiotic resistant propionibacteria in acne: need for policies to modify antibiotic usage', *British Medical Journal*, 306: 55–6, 1993

Chapter 4

1. Bassett, I.B., Pannowitz, D.L., Barnetson, R.S. 'A comparative study of tea-tree oil versus benzyl peroxide in the treatment of acne', *The Medical Journal of Australia*, 153(8): 455–8, 1990

2. El-akawi, Z., Abdel-latif, N., & Abdul-Razzak, K. 'Does the plasma level of vitamin A and E affect acne condition?', *Clinical & Experimental Dermatology*, 31(3): 430–4, May 2006

3. Amer, M., Bahgat, M.R., Tosson, Z., Abdel Mowla M.Y., Amer, K. 'Serum zinc in acne vulgaris', *International Journal of Dermatology*, 21(8): 481–4, October 1982

Chapter 5

1   Acne Support Group survey of members, 1997 (unpublished)

Chapter 7

1   McDougall, M.J., Tan, S.L., Balen, A., Jacobs, H.S. 'A controlled study comparing patients with and without polycystic ovaries undergoing in-vitro fertilisation', *Human Reproduction*, 8: 233–236, 1993

2   Cahill, D. 'PCOS', *Clinical Evidence Handbook*, 80: 620–1, 2009

Chapter 8

1   Berg, M. and Liden, S. 'An epidemiological study of rosacea', *Acta Dermato-Venereologica*, 69: 419–23, 1989

2   Acne Support Group survey of members, 2005 (unpublished)

3   Wilkin, Jonathan MD. 'Standard classification of rosacea: report of the National Rosacea Society Expert Committee on the Classification and Staging of Rosacea', *Journal of the American Academy of Dermatology*, 46(4): 584–7, April 2002

4   Browning, D.J. and Proia, A.D. 'Ocular rosacea', *Survey of Ophthalmology*, 31: 145–58, 1986

Chapter 9

1   Rigopoulos, D. 'Randomised placebo-controlled trial of a flavonoid-rich plant extract-based cream in the treatment of rosacea', *Journal of the European Academy of Dermatology and Venereology*, 19: 564–8, 2005

2   Acne Support Group survey of members, 2005 (unpublished)

Chapter 13

1   Acne Support Group survey of members, 2003 (unpublished)

2   Salamon, M., Chodkiewicz, J., Sysa-Jedrzejowska, A., Wozniacka, A., 'Quality of life assessment of patients with rosacea', *Medical review* 65(9): 385–9, 2008

RESOURCES

Acne.org
A patient-run, US-based organisation that gives a wide range of practical advice and information on all aspects of acne.
www.acne.org

British Association of Dermatologists
The regulatory body for dermatologists in the UK. Learn more about the role and training of UK dermatologists.
www.bad.org.uk; 020 7383 0266

British Red Cross
Provides skin camouflage advice and demonstration, available via appointment with clinics held in hospital dermatology departments.
www.redcross.org.uk; 0844 412 2804

British Association for Hidradenitis Suppurativa
An organisation dedicated to raising awareness and understanding of this painful condition which is linked to acne.
www.bahs.org.uk

British Association of Skin Camouflage
Provides training and comprehensive information on all aspects of skin camouflage, including a contact list of accredited practitioners in your area.
www.skin-camouflage.net; 01254 703107

DermNet NZ
A comprehensive online resource dedicated to every skin condition imaginable.
www.dermnetnz.org

MHRA
The agency responsible for licensing and monitoring licensed medicines. Report unwanted side effects here or discover more about how medicines are monitored.
www.mhra.gov.uk; 020 7084 2000

PCOS UK
The charity for women affected by polycystic ovarian syndrome and campaigns for greater awareness and education into this relatively common condition.
www.pcos-uk.org.uk

Skin Camouflage Network
Represents the National Association of Skin Camouflage Practitioners and offers study days, news and signposting to local practitioners
www.skincamouflagenetwork.org.uk; 07851 073795

Skin Care Campaign
Campaigning organisation for better care and services for people with skin conditions
www.skincarecampaign.org

Books

Acne: The at your fingertips guide by Tim Mitchell and Alison Dudley (Class
    Publishing, 2002)
*PCOS Diet Book: How you can use the nutritional approach to deal with poly-
    cystic ovary syndrome* by Collette Harris and Theresa Cheung (Thorsons,
    2002)
Spotless: The essential guide to getting rid of spots and acne by Elaine Mummery
    (Matador, 2009)

ACKNOWLEDGEMENTS

Many thanks to Ed Seaton, who has trained with the best acne specialists in the UK and is not only an excellent dermatologist, but also a caring and compassionate doctor who really knows his stuff. Other influential dermatologists in the field include the now retired Professor Cunliffe and Dr Alison Layton, both of whom have helped advances in acne and rosacea in a myriad of ways and I would like to take this opportunity to acknowledge their contribution to dermatology. Thank you to Carla Mitchell for her determination to raise the profile of acne and rosacea among her fellow beauty therapists with a dynamic and enthusiastic passion. A lot of my information on skincare and sun protection is down to her knowledge and advice. Thank you also to Nula Bealby, who helped me to bring awareness of the Acne Support Group to millions and for the guidance, knowledge and support she gave to me personally when I felt I was fighting some battles alone. For their patience and love, I would like to thank my husband, Nick, and daughters, Charlotte, Emily, Jess and Lucy.

INDEX